T0215071

Systematic Reviews
TO SUPPORT EVIDENCE-BASED MEDICINE

Authoritative, clear and concise, this award-winning book continues to be an essential text for all medical, surgical and allied health professionals who are seeking a quick and respected guide to systematically reviewing the literature. The third edition features a new chapter on 'Publishing systematic reviews' and numerous new case studies covering the latest developments in the field, including umbrella reviews, reviews of test accuracy, qualitative evidence, prognostic studies, and practice guidelines.

The highly experienced authors, who have each contributed to numerous systematic reviews that have helped form policy and practice, ensure that this practical text, which avoids technical jargon, continues to be the reference of choice for all health professionals undertaking literature reviews, including those specializing in epidemiology and public health.

Systematic Reviews

TO SUPPORT EVIDENCE-BASED MEDICINE

HOW TO APPRAISE, CONDUCT AND PUBLISH REVIEWS

THIRD EDITION

Khalid S. Khan

Beatriz Galindo Distinguished Investigator and Professor of Preventive Medicine and Public Health at the University of Granada, Spain
Researcher of the Spanish Research Network in Epidemiology and Public Health (CIBERESP)

Javier Zamora

Head of the Clinical Biostatistics Unit at Ramon y Cajal University Hospital (IRYCIS), Madrid, Spain
Professor of Biostatistics in Maternal and Perinatal Health at the University of Birmingham, UK
Researcher of the Spanish Research Network in Epidemiology and Public Health (CIBERESP)

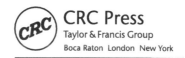

CRC Press
Taylor & Francis Group
Boca Raton London New York

CRC Press is an imprint of the
Taylor & Francis Group, an **Informa** business

Third edition published 2023
by CRC Press
6000 Broken Sound Parkway NW, Suite 300, Boca Raton, FL 33487-2742

and by CRC Press
4 Park Square, Milton Park, Abingdon, Oxon, OX14 4RN

CRC Press is an imprint of Taylor & Francis Group, LLC

Second edition published 2011

ISBN: 9781032114736 (hbk)
ISBN: 9781032114675 (pbk)
ISBN: 9781003220039 (ebk)

DOI: 10.1201/9781003220039

Typeset in Rotis Semi Sans Std
by KnowledgeWorks Global Ltd.

Contents

Preface

Are you about to start working on your first review project? Do you wish to become a published author of a systematic review? Are you embarking on a career in public health, epidemiology or health technology assessment? Are you a clinical teacher interested in discovering the likely educational effects of the courses you deliver? Are you interested in health from the social science perspective? Are you a health professional who wishes to improve the quality of your practice using guidelines? If so, this book is for you.

The first two editions of this book exceeded all expectations. It was commended in the Basis of Medicine category in the BMA Medical Book competition 2003. Commentators found it a clear, useful guide to a potentially off-putting topic that built the confidence of non-statisticians. The *British Journal of Surgery* called it a 'gem'. It recognized that this book stood head and shoulders above other texts on account of its brevity and clarity of prose. It advised readers that if they ever read or wrote systematic reviews, they should read this book first. It was praised for conveying an enthusiasm that made the reader want to conduct a review of their own. Its well-organized materials, logical structured flow, useful worked examples and case studies led to it being recommended to libraries of educational and research institutions concerned with health sciences. It was directed at novice reviewers, and it has been cited hundreds of times, indicating that even seasoned researchers have taken an interest in its contents. With the passage of time, a third edition became imperative. Like its predecessors, this edition describes the main principles behind systematic reviews of healthcare research and provides guidance on how reviews can be appraised, conducted and applied in practice. It adds guidance on how to write up reviews for publication in peer-reviewed journals.

As our healthcare practice and policy increasingly relies on clear and comprehensive summaries of information collated through systematic literature reviews, it is necessary for us to understand how reviews and clinical practice guidelines are produced. You may not be trained in health research methods, but this book will enable you to grasp the principles behind reviewing published literature. In this way, you will be able to critically appraise published systematic reviews and guidelines, and evaluate their inferences and recommendations for application in your practice.

Published reviews and guidelines are not always adequate or sufficient for our needs. Have you ever wondered how you could conduct your own review? The resources required for undertaking reviews are available in a clinical setting. The appointment of clinical librarians, internet access to journals, ease of obtaining papers online and the availability of user-friendly software make it possible for systematic reviews to be conducted by healthcare practitioners and bachelor's or master's degree students. This book highlights the core information necessary for planning, preparing and publishing reviews. It focuses on a clinical readership and new reviewers, not on experienced epidemiologists and statisticians. Using this book, you will be able to initiate your own review and write it up for publication in a peer-reviewed journal.

What is new in this edition of the book? We have widened the scope to go beyond the evaluation of the effectiveness of interventions in healthcare. We demonstrate how reviews can be usefully applied to evaluate qualitative and educational research. We have thoroughly overhauled the section and examples on how to interpret the findings of a review, leading to judicious and credible recommendations for clinical practice. We have added a substantial number of new case studies, providing more worked illustrations of key concepts.

What is totally new in this book is its additional content on how to write up the manuscript of a review for publication. New reviewers just don't have the confidence to go ahead with writing up their reviews. A master's degree student may have undertaken a literature review for preparing their thesis. Their effort is visible in the detailed manuscript, but it is far too wordy for a published article. How can the written work be cut down in size from 50,000 to 3,000 words? This book will take new reviewers through the manuscript writing process so that they can confidently submit a quality manuscript compliant with all reporting guidelines and journals' instructions.

For too many years there has been a mystery surrounding systematic reviews and reviewers. How did they select certain studies and reject others? What did they do to collate the results? How did a bunch of insignificant findings suddenly become significant? How did they capture a very large body of evidence summarized in a succinct published article? You are about to embark on a journey that will demystify these intrigues. Enjoy reading and get your review published.

Khalid S. Khan
Javier Zamora

About the authors

Together we are veterans of over 300 published systematic reviews. Over the years we have worked with healthcare commissioners, clinicians and other decision-makers, producing reviews to inform policy and practice. We have collaborated with other epidemiologists and statisticians to advance methods for undertaking systematic reviews. The two of us work in a clinical academic setting producing, promoting and applying systematic reviews to inform practice. We have supervised many students to undertake graduate and doctoral thesis work based on systematic reviews and to publish their reviews in peer-reviewed journals.

Khalid S. Khan is Professor and Distinguished Investigator in Public Health and Preventive Medicine at the University of Granada, Spain. He has been Professor at the University of Birmingham and the Queen Mary University of London, UK, and Spinoza Professor at the University of Amsterdam, the Netherlands. With an h-index >100, he has published over 150 peer-reviewed systematic review papers collating data from 6415 studies with 68,798,079 participants. He is among the top 2% most influential scientists in the world. He is a clinician, trained in systematic reviews and evidence-based medicine (EBM). Qualified in medical education, he has run journal clubs and other EBM activities, including evidence-supported ward rounds and workshops on critical appraisal. He teaches undergraduates and postgraduates. His Core Outcomes in Women's and Newborn Health (CROWN) initiative was awarded a BMA Strutt and Harper grant to help reduce research waste. He is former Editor of *BJOG*, *EBM-BMJ* and *BMC Med Educ*. In this role, over 10,000 manuscripts have been evaluated for publication under his editorship. He runs an active teaching programme for researchers and reviewers on how to write up manuscripts that editors find acceptable for publication.

Javier Zamora is Professor of Biostatistics at the University of Birmingham, UK, and Head of the Clinical Biostatistics Unit of the Ramon y Cajal Hospital (IRYCIS Research Institute) in Madrid, Spain. He has been Senior Lecturer at the Queen Mary University of London, UK, and Associate Professor at the Complutense University of Madrid, Spain. He is also among the top 2% most influential scientists in the world. He leads a research group of Epidemiology and Public Health within the CIBERESP research excellence network in Spain. He is also Deputy Head of the Madrid Associate Cochrane Centre where he supports the production and dissemination of evidence synthesis activities. He has been involved as a statistician and methodologist in many systematic reviews and meta-analyses which have been published in high-ranking journals such as *Cochrane Database of Systematic Reviews*, *JAMA*, *Annals of Internal Medicine*, *Lancet*, *BMJ* and *PLoS Medicine*. He has been the statistical editor of *BJOG* and has acted as a statistical referee of many peer-reviewed journals. His teaching activities focus on methodology for clinical primary research and for producing evidence syntheses to promote EBM.

We have put this book together because we feel that healthcare professionals have much to gain from reviews and guidelines and, at the same time, reviews and guidelines have much to gain from them. With this book, we hope healthcare practitioners will feel empowered to use reviews effectively, to initiate their own reviews to collate the published literature systematically and to publish their reviews confidently in peer-reviewed journals.

Acknowledgements

No work can ever be completed without the support of many. The authors are grateful to Susan Hahné, Anjum Doshani, Peter J Thompson and Jack Cohen for critical review of earlier versions of this book; Mary Publicover for review of Step 2; Sue O'Meara for review of Case study 3; Elaine Denny for contribution to Case study 5; Sharon Buckley for contribution to Case study 6; Katja Suter for contribution to Case study 7; Luciano Mignini for contribution to Case study 8; Mario Rivera-Izquierdo for review of Case study 9; and Naomi Cano-Ibáñez and Margarita Rojas-Venegas for review of Case study 10. Most of all we are grateful to Jos Kleijnen, Gerd Antes and Regina Kunz for co-authorship of the previous two editions of this book.

Additional contributors

Sharon Buckley
Senior Lecturer in Medical Education, University of Birmingham, UK

Elaine Denny
Professor of Health Sociology, School of Health Sciences, Birmingham City University, UK

Katja Suter
Department of Clinical Research, University of Basel, Switzerland

Luciano Mignini
Medical Investigator, Universidad Nacional de Rosario, Santa Fe, Argentina and Clinical Associate Director, Outreach Research & Innovation Group, Manchester, UK

Abbreviations

BEME	Best Evidence Medical and Health Professions Education Collaboration
CER	Control Event Rate
CI	Confidence Interval
EBM	Evidence-based Medicine
EER	Experimental Event Rate
ES	Effect Size (for continuous data)
GRADE	The Grading of Recommendations Assessment, Development and Evaluation working group
HTA	Health Technology Assessment
IMRaD	Introduction, Methods, Results and Discussion – sections of the manuscript for publication
ITT	Intention-To-Treat analysis
LR	Likelihood Ratio (LR+, LR for positive test result; LR–, LR for negative test result)
MeSH	Medical Subject Heading
NNT	Number Needed to Treat
OR	Odds Ratio (*not to be confused with Boolean operator OR used in searching literature electronically*)
RCT	Randomized Controlled Trial
RD	Risk Difference (or ARR, absolute risk reduction)
RR	Relative Risk
SD	Standard Deviation
SE	Standard Error

Introduction

We hardly ever come across a healthcare journal that does not publish systematic reviews. All disciplines related to medicine and allied health professions, including social science and medical education, rely heavily on reviews for guiding practice and scholarship. What makes them ubiquitous? Reviews provide summaries of evidence contained in a number of individual studies on a specific topic. Research that is relevant to our practice is scattered all over the literature and important research may be published in languages foreign to us. By going through a single review article in our own language, we can get a quick overview of a wide range of evidence on a particular topic. Therefore, we like reviews. They provide us with a way of keeping up to date without the trouble of having to go through the individual studies relevant to our practice. With an ever-increasing number of things to do in our professional lives and not enough time to do them all, who wouldn't find reviews handy? To be honest, even if we had the time and means to identify and appraise relevant individual studies, many of us would still prefer reviews.

Now a word of warning – the manner in which narrative reviews search for studies, collate evidence and generate inferences is often suspect. In the worst cases, the personal interests of the author may drive the whole of the review process and its conclusions. After all, many of the reviews we read are invited commentaries; they are not properly conducted pieces of research. So, how can we be certain that reviews are not misleading us? This is why systematic reviews have come to replace traditional reviews.

Robust systematic reviews of healthcare literature are proper pieces of research. They pose a research question, identify relevant studies, appraise their quality and summarize their results using a scientific methodology. In this way, they differ from traditional reviews and off-the-cuff commentaries produced by 'experts'. More importantly, the recommendations of quality systematic reviews, instead of reflecting personal views of 'experts', are based on balanced inferences generated from the collated evidence.

This book describes the principles behind systematically reviewing the published literature on healthcare and related subjects. Using this book, readers should be able to confidently appraise a review for its quality and interpret its findings, as well as initiate and publish one of their own.

A **systematic review** is a research article that identifies relevant studies, appraises their quality and summarizes their results using a scientific methodology to address a research question.

The term **meta-analysis** is not synonymous with a systematic review. It is only a part of the review. It is a statistical technique for combining the results of a number of individual studies to produce a summary result. Beware, some publications called meta-analyses are not systematic reviews. Note that a systematic review could exist without a meta-analysis but the opposite could not happen.

From here onwards, whenever this book uses the term **review**, it will mean a **systematic review**, using these terms interchangeably. Reviews should never be done in any other way different than systematically.

Meta-synthesis is the synthesis of existing qualitative research findings on a specific research question. This does not involve meta-analysis.

Evidence-based medicine (EBM) is the judicious use of current best evidence in making decisions about healthcare. **Systematic reviews** provide strong evidence to underpin EBM or evidence-based practice.

Evidence synthesis

Evidence synthesis is the general term used to describe a systematic approach to collating relevant evidence from the published literature for addressing a research question. A systematic review to scientifically answer a clearly formulated question deploying a meta-analysis is the queen of the various types of evidence syntheses that exist. The logic of systematically reviewing the literature is nowadays applied in a wide variety of ways leading to such a plethora of published reviews on a topic that a reader can easily become confused. We give a little orientation for novice reviewers.

When a review is undertaken using a systematic approach but without a clearly formulated question, the evidence synthesis is called a **scoping review**. It is used to map the existing evidence to delineate the main themes and the related knowledge gaps. It can serve as a precursor to a systematic review, helping to define the components of its structured question.

A **rapid review** is a systematic review undertaken with an urgency to synthesize evidence. The idea is to produce a review over a short time frame while maintaining scientific rigor. As we all know well, things done in a hurry with limited resources (time is a key resource in review projects) may sacrifice the desired quality as shortcuts tend to be inherently risky.

A systematic review may become outdated as soon as it is published, particularly in a field where research is actively taking place. The emergence of new individual studies should trigger an update of the existing review. The policy for updating completed reviews is not standard, but **living systematic reviews** have recently risen to the fore with the aim to keep the review findings updated through continuous effort. This approach is particularly useful in developing scenarios such as a new pandemic. Artificial intelligence techniques are being developed in computer sciences to assist reviewers to undertake rapid and living reviews.

At the time of writing, it is estimated that over 20,000 systematic reviews are published annually, i.e. around 55 every day. Thus, on a given topic, there might already be many reviews available. In this situation, a review of reviews may usefully collate the evidence, critically appraising the quality of the existing reviews and drawing inferences from a synthesis of their findings. Such a review is called an **umbrella review**. The inference of an umbrella review might well be that a new systematic review is needed.

> **Evidence synthesis** is a systematic approach to collating relevant evidence to address a research question. **Systematic review**, an evidence synthesis to scientifically answer a clearly formulated question, is just one of the various types of evidence syntheses. Among other evidence synthesis types are included: scoping review, rapid review, living systematic review, umbrella review, guidelines, etc.

> An **umbrella review** is an evidence synthesis in the form of a review of systematic reviews on a topic. Following a critical appraisal of all the relevant reviews, it might provide underpinning evidence for evidence-based practice or it might conclude that there is a need for conducting a new review.

Critically appraising systematic reviews

More and more healthcare policy is being based on clear and comprehensive summaries of information collated through systematic reviews of the relevant literature. Umbrella reviews frequently underpin guidance documents. So, in the current day and age, evidence-based practice requires more than just a critical appraisal of individual studies. Clinical practice guidelines are a prime example of how systematic reviews have come to occupy a pivotal role in our professional lives.

Systematic reviews may represent a quantum leap in review methodology. However, we should not have blind faith. Reviews, just like individual studies, can be of a variable quality. There are numerous examples of poor-quality systematic reviews published in top healthcare journals and of inferior guidelines produced by professional bodies. Hence, there is a potential for misleading inferences even among apparently robust reviews. Therefore, it is necessary for us, as healthcare practitioners, to acquire a deeper understanding of the principles behind systematic reviews. Although we may only have basic knowledge of health research methods and consider the task of appraising reviews onerous, with this book, readers will be able to grasp the processes and pitfalls of systematically reviewing the literature and discriminate between robust and not-so-robust reviews more easily.

We can identify existing reviews to support our practice by searching the resources shown in Box 0.1. Once relevant reviews have been identified, the quality of their methods should be appraised, their evidence should be examined and their findings should be assessed for applicability in practice. Sometimes umbrella reviews may give an overview of all the available systematic reviews on a topic. Examples of how to appraise and use findings from existing reviews are shown in the Case studies in Section B of this book. When drawing on reviews to support our practice, we will occasionally become painfully aware that relevant reviews do not exist. Often there will be reviews but on critical appraisal, they will be found lacking in quality. When you can't find a review that meets your needs, why not initiate a new one?

Conducting a systematic review

Internet access to literature searching, the ability to obtain articles either electronically or through interlibrary loans, user-friendly software for meta-analysis, etc. all make systematic reviewing possible. As these resources are increasingly available in a clinical setting, undertaking systematic reviews has become a realistic option for healthcare practitioners. But why should practitioners undertake reviews?

There is no shortage of reasons for undertaking one's own review. One may wish to conduct reviews for supporting evidence-based practice, personal professional development, informing clinical policy, publishing in a peer-reviewed journal, writing the background to a research thesis or preparing a presentation at a conference, a technical report or an invited commentary.

However, there should be no need to reinvent the wheel. Existing reviews should be used to their full potential. Up-to-date good quality reviews may already contain all the information needed.

Guidelines are systematically developed statements to assist practitioners and patients in making decisions about specific clinical situations. They should ideally, but don't always, use evidence from **systematic reviews** to generate recommendations.

What is involved in the identification, appraisal and application of evidence summarized in reviews?

Framing questions
↓
Identifying relevant reviews
↓
Assessing the quality of the review and its evidence
↓
Summarizing the evidence
↓
Interpreting the findings

The **Cochrane Collaboration**, established in 1993, is an international network of people helping healthcare providers, policymakers, patients, their advocates and carers make well-informed decisions about healthcare by preparing, updating and promoting the accessibility of Cochrane Reviews.

Box 0.1 Selected sources of systematic reviews

The Internet search engines capture reviews whenever one writes the keywords systematic review or meta-analysis in the search box. There are more systematic reviews around than one might think!

Prospero (www.crd.york.ac.uk/prospero) is a database of systematic reviews that have been prospectively registered prior to commencing the review.

The Cochrane Library (www.cochranelibrary.com) has several databases of published and ongoing systematic reviews. The library contained 11,015 completed reviews and review protocols combined at the time of writing.

International HTA database (database.inahta.org) contains reports of health technology assessments (HTA) produced by members of the International Network of Agencies for Health Technology Assessment (INAHTA) and other healthcare technology agencies. At the time of writing, HTA database contained 17,701 records, mostly systematic review based.

General electronic databases (also see Box 2.2) like PubMed permit searches to be limited to systematic reviews or meta-analyses simply by clicking on the options provided under article type. At the time of writing, there were 216,519 systematic review citations included in PubMed. CINAHL, EMBASE, PsycLIT and other databases may be searched for reviews by applying one of the many available systematic review search filters (a combination of text words, indexing terms and subject headings that captures the relevant article type).

Online systematic review repositories (e.g. ksrevidence.com or epistemonikos.org) continuously update searches to collate published systematic reviews, meta-analyses and healthcare technology assessments. KSR Evidence had 206,236 systematic reviews at the time of writing.

Guidelines International Network (g-i-n.net) contains >6000 guidelines from 96 groups in 76 countries.

Websites are constantly changing. The internet addresses provided in this book were obtained during searches in January 2022.

When reviews on a specific topic do not exist, are not up to date or are of a poor quality, our options are: ask 'experts' for advice, appraise available primary studies or conduct a systematic review.

We realize that 'expert' opinions may not be evidence based and they may be unacceptable to others – for every 'expert', there is an equal and opposite 'expert'. We know that appraisal of individual studies available to us will not provide information on the complete picture. Isn't this the point where we want to start a new review? Many reviews commence in this way and when they are published, everyone can benefit from them. Conducting a new systematic review will take effort, but not everything that is worthwhile is easy.

When undertaking research projects for educational assignments, we (or at least our supervisors) should be aware that non-systematic reviews are increasingly less acceptable. Where do we go next? We should do our own systematic review. As academics in the health professions (without advanced epidemiology and statistics training), we may be used to publishing editorials, opinions and commentaries. We are now under pressure from journal editors to be more systematic in our approach. Why not try a systematic review for the next commentary? We may feel inhibited as the knowledge or skills required for initiating such reviews may not be within our grasp. Help is in our hands. This book provides the core information necessary for planning and initiating reviews of healthcare literature.

This book focuses primarily on a clinical readership and first-time reviewers, not on seasoned epidemiologists, social scientists, educationalists and statisticians. This book will enable readers to initiate reviews without relying on professional reviewers and will also give advice about when to seek professional input in difficult areas. Considering the nature of work involved in the various Steps of a review, it is advisable to find co-reviewers to join in early. First-time reviewers might want to attend a local workshop or course on systematic reviews. There are many online resources and webinars – why not register for an online training event to supplement the learning acquired through this book.

Cochrane Reviews are systematic reviews of primary research in healthcare and health policy. They investigate the effects of interventions (literally meaning to intervene to modify an outcome) for prevention, treatment and rehabilitation. They also assess the accuracy of tests.

How this book is structured

This book will help readers to understand the principles of systematic reviews. In the discourse that follows, there is a step-by-step explanation of the review process. There are just five Steps. This book provides guidance for each Step of a review with examples from published reviews. Many examples are followed through the different Steps so that we will be able to see the link between the Steps. In addition, the application of the theory is illustrated through Case studies. Each case consists of a scenario requiring evidence from reviews, a demonstration of review methods and a proposed resolution of the scenario. Insight into critical appraisal and conducting a systematic review can be gained by working through the various Steps, examples and Case studies.

If we have made up our mind to initiate a review, we should first produce a brief outline (or a protocol) of the project, giving some background information and a specification of the problem to be addressed along with the methodology to be used in the review. This, once discussed and agreed among the review team, should be prospectively registered before commencing the review work. Throughout the various Steps of the review, the protocol will remind us where we are coming from and what direction we need to take, avoiding distractions and keeping us on track. It will also provide a document that could be developed for peer review. Such a well-developed review protocol may be submitted to a peer-reviewed journal for publication as an article.

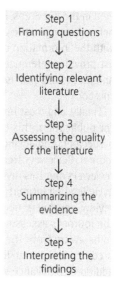

Step 1
Framing questions
↓
Step 2
Identifying relevant literature
↓
Step 3
Assessing the quality of the literature
↓
Step 4
Summarizing the evidence
↓
Step 5
Interpreting the findings

Registration of the review with a relevant Review Group of the Cochrane, Best Evidence Medical and Health Professions Education (BEME) or other collaborations that offer the opportunity to obtain input into the protocol is a good way forward. Alternatively, the review protocol may be uploaded on a prospective registration site, posted on an open science online forum or on the reviewer's own website to obtain comments from interested parties, but input from visitors to the site may be variable. Realistically, we have a much better chance of getting a professional to comment on the protocol quickly if we ask a colleague experienced in reviewing.

This book will be a useful companion in protocol development as well as throughout the five Steps in the review process:

- First, the problems to be addressed have to be specified in the form of well-structured questions (Step 1). This is a key step, as all other aspects of the review follow directly from the questions.
- Second, thorough literature searches have to be conducted to identify potentially relevant studies which can shed light on the questions (Step 2). This is an essential feature that makes a review systematic.
- Third, the quality of the selected studies is assessed to appraise their scientific rigour (Step 3).
- Fourth, the evidence is summarized concerning study features, participants and data, and results (Step 4). When feasible and appropriate, statistical analysis (e.g. meta-analysis) helps in collating results.
- Finally, inferences and recommendations for practice are generated by interpreting and exploring the clinical relevance and trustworthiness of the findings (Step 5).

The key points about appraisal and conduct of reviews are summarized at the end of each Step in Section A of this book. The Case studies in Section B illustrate the application of the reviewing theory that is covered in the five Steps. Readers may prefer to assimilate the review theory before turning to the Case studies or they may read them in conjunction with the information contained in the first section. A suggested reading list provides references to direct readers to other texts for theoretical and methodological issues that are beyond the core material covered in this book.

Finally, and most importantly for people undertaking reviews to write for publication, this book includes tips and tricks on how to prepare a succinct, convincing manuscript for submission to a peer-reviewed journal. Reviewers frequently face rejection by journal editors and peer reviewers and this invariably wastes time in the rejection–resubmission cycle leading ultimately to publication. In addition to undertaking the review, reviewers need to understand the manuscript structure and the journal's assessments in the publication process. Reviewers need to be aware from the outset that the article structure and length are predetermined and fixed according to the journal's instructions. In addition, compliance with a reporting checklist will likely be mandatory.

The **Best Evidence in Medical and Health Professions Education (BEME)** Collaboration is committed to the promotion of BEME through the dissemination and production of systematic reviews of medical education. An additional objective is the creation of a culture of BEME amongst teachers, institutions and national bodies.

IMRaD is an acronym that refers to the section headings used in writing the main manuscript text, i.e. I-Introduction, M-Methods, R-Results, a-and, D-Discussion, of a systematic review paper for submission to a peer-reviewed journal. At the end of each Step in Section A, this book provides guidance to review authors for drafting text within these headings.

To facilitate efficient drafting of the manuscript, we provide specific advice for review authors at the end of each Step in Section A of this book. We share many unwritten rules that will hopefully increase the probability of a review paper being accepted for publication on its first submission to a journal.

The guidance in this book is pitched at a level suitable for users of systematic reviews and for novice reviewers. It should not be seen as providing a 'set menu' for appraising and undertaking systematic reviews. What it offers is a range of 'à la carte' guidance, which can be applied flexibly depending on the review question and context.

This book will focus in Section A on the five Steps for systematic reviews of reported research examining the effects of *interventions* or *exposures* on *outcomes*. In Section B, its Case studies will also cover reviews examining test accuracy, medical education, qualitative research, etc.

Key points about this book

- This book will enable readers to confidently appraise published reviews for their quality, as well as to initiate and publish their own reviews.
- It describes the main principles behind systematically reviewing published literature on the effects of healthcare, focusing on a readership of healthcare professionals.
- It includes a step-by-step explanation of how to appraise and conduct reviews along with illustrative examples and Case studies.
- Key points about critical appraisal and conduct of a review are summarized at the end of each Step.
- Writing tips are provided for review authors on how to convert the extensive review work undertaken into a succinct manuscript for submission to a peer-reviewed journal.

Section A: *Steps of a systematic review*

This section provides a step-by-step explanation of what is involved in carrying out a systematic review. There are just five Steps. For each Step, the basic principles of a review are explained, using examples from published review articles. Many examples are followed through the different steps so that readers will be able to see the link between the various stages of a review.

Step 1: Framing questions for a review

Step 2: Identifying relevant literature

Step 3: Assessing the quality of the literature

Step 4: Summarizing the evidence

Step 5: Interpreting the findings

DOI: 10.1201/9781003220039-1

Step 1: *Framing questions for a review*

Step 1
Framing questions
↓
Step 2
Identifying relevant literature
↓
Step 3
Assessing the quality of the literature
↓
Step 4
Summarizing the evidence
↓
Step 5
Interpreting the findings

Systematic reviews are carried out to generate answers to focused questions about healthcare and related issues. The key to a successful review project lies in the reviewer's ability to be precise and specific when stating the problems to be addressed in the review. This is a critical part of the review because, as will become apparent in subsequent Steps, all other aspects of the review flow directly from the questions framed initially. If in a particular review a question cannot be precisely formulated, stating this transparently is an essential feature of a good review. In this Step, we will examine the question formulation process in detail, briefly look at the thinking required to examine the potential impact of variations in the different components of a review question and consider the options available for prospective registration of a review project.

1.1 An approach to formulating questions

Formulating questions is not as easy as it may sound. A structured approach to framing questions, which uses four components or facets, may be used. These components include the *participants*, *interventions* or *exposures*, *outcomes* related to the problem posed in the review and the *designs* of studies that are suitable for addressing it. We can see the relationship between the various question components in the comparative study in Box 1.1.

After looking through Box 1.1, the formulation of questions will probably seem like a daunting task to new reviewers. We may begin to have second thoughts, but we should not give up – help is at hand. This chapter will take us through the question formulation process so that our review can have just the right start. It is well recognized that even quite experienced clinicians don't always find it easy to frame questions for evidence-based practice, so new reviewers can also expect to have a rough ride during the initial stages of their reviews. It will take some effort, but its value will be realized soon, as the rest of the review will flow directly and efficiently from the framed questions.

Most serious reviewers devote a substantial amount of time and effort to getting the questions right before embarking on a review. They may even carry out a scoping review to inform the development of their systematic review question. They do this because they want to avoid having to change questions later on during the course of conducting the review. We should also pay a great deal of attention to detail in this Step. If there is any difficulty in figuring out the components of questions, we should

Question components
- The participants
- The interventions or exposures
- The outcomes
- The study designs

Free-form question: It describes the query for which one seeks an answer through a review in simple language (however vague).

DOI: 10.1201/9781003220039-2

Box 1.1 Framing structured questions for systematic reviews

Question components

- The participants — A succinct description of a group of people or patients, their clinical problem and the healthcare setting.
- The interventions or exposures — The main action(s) being considered, e.g. treatments, processes of care, social intervention, educational intervention, tests, etc., or exposures being measured, e.g. risk factors, smoking, dietary practices, etc.
- The outcomes — The clinical changes desired in health state (morbidity, mortality) over a specified time period or duration of follow-up.
- The study design — The appropriate ways to recruit participants or patients in a research study, give them interventions or measure their exposures, follow them up and evaluate their outcomes.

Relationship between the question components in a comparative study

A comparative study assesses the effect of an intervention using comparison groups. For example, it may allocate *participants* from a relevant group of people or patients (with or without randomization) to alternative *interventions* or *exposures* and follow them up to determine the effect of the *interventions* or *exposures* on the *outcome*.

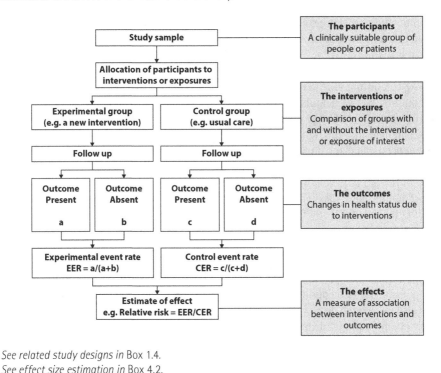

See related study designs in Box 1.4.
See effect size estimation in Box 4.2.

first write them down in the free form. We can then reconstruct the free-form question into a structured format as exemplified in Box 1.2.

We should think of *participants* as a description of the group of people or patients about whom evidence is being sought in the review. Imagine *interventions* as the actions or the alternatives being considered for the *participants*. *Outcomes* are measures of what the *participants* want to achieve from the *interventions*, e.g. avoiding illness or death. Finally, we should think of how a worthwhile study could be *designed* to examine the effect of the *interventions*. For example, by comparing *outcomes* between groups of *participants* with and without

Structured question: Reviewers convert free-form questions into a clear and explicit format using a structured approach (see Box 1.2). This makes the query potentially answerable through existing relevant studies.

Box 1.2 Some example questions

Nature of question: Clinical effectiveness

Free-form question: Which of the many available antimicrobial products improve the healing of chronic wounds?

Structured question

● The participants	In adults with various forms of chronic wounds in an ambulatory setting ....
● The interventions	.... would systemic or topical antimicrobial preparations ....
● The outcomes	.... improve wound healing at 3 months?
● The study design	A comparative study that allocates subjects with chronic wounds to alternative therapeutic interventions of interest and determines the effect of the interventions on wound healing (e.g. randomized controlled trial) (*see Box 1.4*).

See Case study 3 for a related review.

Nature of question: Aetiology

Free-form question: Is exposure to benzodiazepines in pregnancy associated with malformations in the newborn baby?

Structured question

● The participants	In pregnant women ....
● The exposures	.... does exposure to benzodiazepines during early pregnancy ....
● The outcomes	.... cause malformations in the newborn baby?
● The study designs	● A study that recruits women in early pregnancy, assesses their exposure to benzodiazepines, follows them up and examines their newborn babies to compare the rates of malformations among women with exposure and those without (cohort study).
	● A study that identifies women who have given birth to a child with malformation and those who have given birth to a healthy child, and compares their exposures to benzodiazepines in early pregnancy (case-control study) (*see Box 1.4*).

See Box 4.6 for a related meta-analysis.

Nature of question: Test accuracy

Free-form question: Among postmenopausal women with abnormal vaginal bleeding, does a pelvic ultrasound scan exclude uterine cancer accurately?

Structured question

● The participants	In postmenopausal women, within a community setting, with vaginal bleeding ....
● The test	.... does a uterine ultrasound scan test accurately confirm or refute ....
● The reference standard	.... the histological diagnosis of uterine cancer?
● The study design	A study that recruits women participants referred from a community clinic, uses the test (scan) and applies a reference standard investigation to confirm or refute the presence of cancer (histology) and determines the accuracy with which the test identifies cancer (*see Box C4.3*).

See Case study 4 for a related review.

Nature of question: Qualitative research

Free-form question: How does the experience of endometriosis impact women's lives?

Structured question

● The participants	In women with a confirmed diagnosis of endometriosis....
● The intervention	.... how does observation or treatment....
● The outcomes	.... affect pain, social relationships and self-image?
● The study design	A study that narrates subjective experiences (*see Box C5.3*).

See Case study 5 for a related review.

Nature of question: Education

Free-form question: How does the use of portfolios affect student learning in undergraduate medical and nursing education?

Structured question

● The participants	Among undergraduate nursing or medical students ....
● The intervention	.... does a 'portfolio', defined as a collection of evidence of student learning, a learning journal or diary or a combination of these two elements ....
● The outcomes	.... improve knowledge and skills?
● The study design	A study that evaluates the educational outcomes and effects of portfolios.

See Case study 6 for a related review.

the *intervention*, the effect of the *intervention* may be assessed in terms of illness avoided.

The point about question formulation is that a structured approach should be used. The structure outlined in Box 1.1 should never become a 'straight jacket', and it may be modified to meet the needs of our free-form question, depending on the nature of our interest in healthcare. For example, in epidemiology, the questions may be about aetiology. We can easily substitute the component *interventions* with *exposure* and frame the questions in terms of how *outcomes* might be different in *participants* exposed or not exposed to certain agents or risk factors (Box 1.2). For questions about the accuracy of screening or diagnostic tests, we might substitute the component *interventions* with *tests* and *outcomes* with *reference standards* against which the accuracy of the *test* will be measured (Box 1.2). In this way, the proposed structure is versatile and adaptable for a wide range of question types.

At the end of this exercise, if we are unable to define a structured question, we have the option of carrying out a scoping review. This will be publishable as a review article in its own right and will help to define the various components of the focused question for a future systematic review.

1.2 Variations in participants, interventions and outcomes

Once the way in which questions are structured is understood (Box 1.1), we should be able to see that systematic reviews are analyses of existing studies within a given set of *participants*, *interventions* and *outcomes* (Box 1.2). We may have started with some scepticism about framing our question in this way; however, with the realization that different *participants*, *interventions* and *outcomes* exist within our free-form question, we are likely to end up with many more than one question. If we have not, we should look hard to see if we haven't missed something. There is bound to be some variation within each of our question components. This is critical – even in a straightforward question about antimicrobials for chronic wounds (Box 1.2), it should be clear that there are many types of chronic wounds (*participants*), antimicrobials (*interventions*) and ways of measuring wound healing (*outcomes*) (Box 1.3).

It is important to seriously consider how *participants*, *interventions* and *outcomes* might vary among existing studies. Such differences are important in defining study selection criteria (Step 2) and planning the tabulation of findings (Steps 4 and 5). They are also relevant in understanding the reasons for variation in the effects of *interventions* from study to study (Step 4) and in exploring the strength of the evidence to gauge the applicability of the findings (Step 5).

Section A of this book will focus mainly on questions relating to the **quantitative** effects of *interventions* (therapy, prevention, social care, etc.) or *exposures* (environmental agents, risk factors, etc.) in the context of **comparative** *study designs*.

Section B of this book, the Case studies, will also cover other types of systematic reviews including syntheses of qualitative and educational research.

A **scoping review** is a systematic review without a clearly formulated question. It follows the methods outlined in Section A of this book delineating the features of the literature on a given topic. This way, following publication, it helps to define the various components of the focused question for a future systematic review.

Box 1.3 Framing questions for reviews: Variations in *participants, interventions, outcomes* and *study designs*

Nature of question: Clinical effectiveness

Free-form question: Which of the many available antimicrobial products improve the healing of chronic wounds?

Structured question *(expanded from Box 1.2)*

● The participants	Adults with various forms of chronic wounds:	● Diabetic ulcers ● Venous ulcers ● Pressure ulcers
● The interventions	Antimicrobial preparations: *Versus* Comparator:	● Systemic preparations ● Topical preparations *Versus* ● Other preparations
● The outcomes	Various measures to quantify the improvement in a critical outcome 'wound healing' with various timings of assessments:	● Outcome measured directly: Complete healing, amputation due to wound complications ● Outcome measured indirectly: The number of dressings per week, wound area remaining, healing scores and reduction in histologically documented inflammation
● The study design	Experimental and observational studies *(see Box 1.4)*:	● Randomized controlled trials ● Experimental studies without randomization ● Cohort studies with concurrent controls

See Case study 3 for a related review.

Free-form question: Do home visits improve the health of elderly people?

Structured question

● The participants	Elderly people in various age groups:	● Young-old ● Middle age-old ● Old-old
● The interventions	Home visits: *Versus* Comparator:	● Intensive assessments ● Frequent assessments *Versus* ● Usual care
● The outcomes	Various measures to quantify health and health resource use:	● Critical outcome measured directly: Mortality ● Critical outcome measured directly: Functional status ● Important outcome measured directly: Nursing home admissions
● The study design	Experimental studies *(see Box 1.4)*:	● Randomized controlled trials ● Experimental studies without randomization

See Box 4.5 for a related meta-analysis.

Free-form question: Do antibiotics improve children's outcomes in otitis media?

Structured question

● The participants	Children with otitis media:	● Various age groups
● The interventions	Antibiotics: *Versus* Comparator:	● Different preparations *Versus* ● Placebo or no treatment
● The outcomes	Various measures to quantify health:	● Critical outcome measured directly: Eardrum perforation ● Important outcome measured directly: Pain ● Important outcome measured directly: Adverse effects
● The study design	Experimental studies (*see Box 1.4*):	● Randomized controlled trials ● Experimental studies without randomization

See Boxes 5.2 and 5.3 for a related review.

Nature of question: Clinical and cost-effectiveness

Free-form question: To what extent is the risk of post-operative infection reduced by antimicrobial prophylaxis in patients undergoing hip replacement and is it worth the costs?

Structured question

● The participants	Patients undergoing hip replacement:	● Various types of procedures
● The interventions	Antimicrobial prophylaxis: *Versus* Comparator:	● Various types of antibiotics *Versus* ● Placebo ● No antibiotics
● The outcomes	Clinical: Economic:	● Post-operative infection ● Cost per infection prevented
● The study design	Clinical: Economic:	● Experimental studies (*see Box 1.4*) ● Cost-effectiveness analyses

See Box 3.4 also.

Nature of question: Comparison of beneficial and harmful outcomes

Free-form question: Which rennin-system inhibitor is better in treating hypertension and is it worth the potential harms?

Structured question

● The participants	Patients with hypertension:	● Various co-morbidities
● The interventions	Angiotensin receptor blockers:	● Various types

	Versus	*Versus*
	Angiotensin converting enzyme inhibitors (avoiding comparison with placebo):	• Various types
• The outcomes	Clinical:	• Critical beneficial outcome measured directly: Mortality, major cardiovascular events and successful monotherapy
		• Important adverse outcomes measured directly: Cough and withdrawals
• The study design	Mixture of designs (*see Box 1.4*):	• Experimental studies for beneficial effects
		• Experimental and observational studies for adverse effects

See Case study 7 for a related review.

Thus, the conclusions of individual studies and reviews may vary depending on differences in the characteristics of their *participants*, the types of their *interventions* and the ways of measurement of *outcomes*. These issues are examined in detail later on in the book. Here we briefly examine their implications when framing questions.

1.2.1 Variations in participants

Participant characteristics may vary between studies with respect to patients' age and sex, the severity of illness, the presence of coexisting illnesses, etc. For instance, when the effect of home visits is studied among elderly people (Box 1.3), the *intervention* is more effective among young-old rather than old-old people (Box 4.5).

1.2.2 Variations in interventions

The *intervention* features such as the intensity, additional routine care, etc. may also be associated with variable effects. For example, among elderly people, home visits are more effective if multidimensional assessments are used and follow-up is frequent (Box 4.5). Defining the comparator is a critical element. If we wish to compare drug A *versus* drug C, we should be clear about this. The literature may only provide studies comparing drug A *versus* B and drug C *versus* B. This literature will permit an indirect comparison of drug A *versus* C, with drug B being the common comparator. In Case study 1, the question is formulated to compare vitamin D supplementation alone *versus* vitamin D in combination with calcium. They are each compared to placebo in head-to-head comparisons. Using placebo as a common control, it is possible to indirectly compare vitamin D supplementation alone *versus* vitamin D in combination with calcium (Case study 1).

1.2.3 Variations in outcomes

Definition, measurement and delineation of the importance of *outcomes* are vast research subjects in their own right. When framing questions for reviews, we need to identify all clinically relevant *outcomes*, which will help in examining the success or failure of the *interventions*. We should aim to specify the optimal methods and timing of *outcome* measurement. For example, when measuring the effect of an infertility treatment, the desired *outcome* is pregnancy, but how should it be measured? A urinary pregnancy test in early pregnancy, an ultrasound of the uterus in mid pregnancy and the live birth of a healthy baby are possible ways in which the presence or absence of *outcome* may be recorded over a specified duration of follow-up. Variation in the timing of the assessment of the *participants* with respect to *outcomes* can be an important source of heterogeneity. In Case study 3 concerning wound healing, the timing of *outcome* assessment varied between 2 and 20 weeks (Box C3.5). During our review, it may become apparent that existing studies have not properly measured *outcomes* that were critical and important. Identification of these deficiencies in existing studies is important by itself for transparency in reviews.

A relevant *outcome* is one that directly measures issues of importance to the participants. Often these data cannot be easily acquired, and there may be a tendency, both among reviewers and readers, to become interested in intermediate, surrogate or proxy *outcome* measurements. For example, when we are really interested in discovering the effect of fluoride therapy in preventing fractures, we might be tempted to investigate bone mineral content as a surrogate *outcome*, as it would be easier to obtain information about this. How misleading such an approach can be is demonstrated in a randomized controlled trial (*N Engl J Med* 1990; **322**: 802-9, doi: 10.1056/NEJM199003223221203); bone density increased significantly (10–35% at different skeletal sites as compared to placebo) among the participants treated with fluorides; however, there was a nearly three-fold increase in non-vertebral fractures (placebo 24 fractures during 325 person-years of follow-up *versus* fluorides 72 fractures during 310 person-years of follow-up, relative risk 3.2, 95% confidence interval 1.8–5.6, $p = 0.01$), which was unexpected. This makes it evident that conclusions from research based on surrogate *outcomes* are likely to be weak when it comes to making decisions in practice. As we delineate in Step 5, the strength and weakness of evidence should be evaluated separately for each outcome, even when data come from the same studies. Therefore, it is crucial that *outcomes* are set out in detail at the outset of a review project. Patient and public involvement is now expected to be an obligatory part of research as consumer and citizen engagement in science is rightly becoming standard. Lay input can be formally sought in the choice of *outcomes* when framing the review question. Published core *outcomes* sets, a grouping of critical

Clinically relevant *outcomes* directly measure what is critical and important to patients in terms of how they feel, what their function is and whether they survive.

Surrogate *outcome* measurements substitute for direct outcome measures. They include physiological variables or measures of subclinical disease. To be valid, the surrogate must be statistically correlated with the clinically relevant outcome.

Core *outcomes* are a group of critical and important outcomes for which there is consensus that they should be measured and reported. Systematic reviews are used to create a long list of outcomes which is then reduced to a core *outcomes* set through surveys collating evaluations of patients and practitioners.

and important *outcomes* on which consensus has emerged through surveys of patients and practitioners, offer an excellent starting point for delineating review questions.

When considering the *outcomes* for a review question, we should think about what we mean by health. Is it just the absence of illness or disease? This section of the book mainly focuses on quantitative morbidity or mortality *outcomes*. In the next section, we also demonstrate how reviews collate evidence on *outcomes* used in qualitative and educational research (Case studies 5 and 6). Policymakers frequently consider the question of how to achieve optimal *outcomes* with the smallest input of resources. This allows us to discover whether the investment in *interventions* is likely to be worthwhile. In this situation, *outcomes* need to focus on the costs of providing healthcare in addition to clinical *outcomes* (Box 1.3). We will not cover these value-for-money issues much beyond framing the questions. Health technology assessments, frequently underpinned by systematic reviews, report on both the costs and the consequences of *interventions*.

1.3 Variations in study designs

Let us turn our attention to *study design*, the fourth component of a review question (Box 1.1). For a given set of *participants, interventions* and *outcomes*, reviews will provide summaries of existing studies that used different research *designs* (Box 1.2). Why is *design* so important? *Design* of a study determines the validity of the observed effects, i.e. our confidence that the results of a study are likely to approximate to the 'truth' for the participants studied depends on the soundness of its *design*. In this way, *design* serves as a basic marker of study quality. Its importance cannot be emphasized enough. Ultimately the strength of a review's inferences depends on the integrity of the *designs* of the available studies.

Some reviewers consider certain *study designs* to be superior because they feel that the *design* has an inherent value in itself. For example, they may focus exclusively on randomized studies when conducting reviews. Such a view ignores the fact that addressing different types of questions may require the use of different *study designs*. As an example, a question about the accuracy of a test would require a *study design* that prospectively (without randomization) recruits all eligible *participants*, employs the *test* and the *reference standard* investigation to confirm or refute the presence of disease and determines the accuracy with which the test correctly identifies disease (Case study 4). Assessment of long-term or rare *outcomes*, particularly when examining the safety of *interventions* (Case study 2), would be more suited to an observational *design*, not an experimental study. For example, cohort and case-control studies, not randomized trials, would evaluate the effect of *exposure* to benzodiazepines in pregnancy on rare malformations in the newborn baby (Box 5.2).

Even for questions concerning the effectiveness of *interventions*, where randomized trials are generally preferred, it might be difficult to justify a restriction to using randomized studies only. This may be

Valid results are said to be unbiased. **Bias** either exaggerates or underestimates the 'true' effect of an *intervention* or *exposure*.

The **quality** of a study depends on the degree to which its *design*, conduct and analysis minimize **biases**.

Effectiveness is the extent to which an *intervention* (therapy, prevention, diagnosis, screening, education, social care, etc.) produces beneficial *outcomes* under ordinary day-to-day circumstances. In contrast, **efficacy** focuses on the performance of *interventions* under ideal circumstances.

particularly true when such studies are unethical. Sometimes there is just a dearth of randomized studies. For example, in the review on antimicrobials for chronic wounds (Case study 3), despite a comprehensive search, only four clearly randomized studies could be found, so other *designs* had to be included. On the other hand, in Case study 2, where the review considered the safety of water fluoridation, no randomized studies had been published, so it became necessary to consider various other *designs*. Effects of educational interventions are often studied using a range of *designs* (Case study 6). For the evaluation of harmful *outcomes* that are rare, observational design is frequently included in reviews (Case study 7). Sometimes a review may consider a number of separate but related questions. For example, if a review is to include an assessment of efficiency in addition to effectiveness, then *study designs* for economic evaluation will also be required (Box 1.3). Thus, it might be necessary to consider different *designs* simultaneously in some review questions. This multiplicity of *designs* has implications for study quality assessment (Step 3), synthesis (Step 4) and interpretation of findings (Step 5).

> **Efficiency** (cost-effectiveness) is the extent to which the balance between input (costs) and output (*outcomes*) of *interventions* represents value for money.

Insistence on randomized studies, ignoring other types of evidence, might paralyze reviewers as such reviews might never find any studies. Often because of ethical or technical reasons, the best possible evidence can only be obtained from observational studies. When faced with having to make decisions for practice, using the best available evidence is likely to be better than not using any evidence at all. We will need to explore the nature of our questions (effectiveness, aetiology, efficiency, accuracy, prognosis, etc.) and the different ways of addressing the specific issues concerning *participants, interventions* and *outcomes* before us. Then we should select the *study designs* that are likely to provide the most valid answers and develop a hierarchy of *study designs* suitable for our review. This approach will help us define inclusion and exclusion criteria for selecting studies of a minimum acceptable quality (Step 2). Once studies have been included in a review, a detailed assessment of their quality (Step 3) and results (Step 4) will be required to gauge the strength of the evidence (Step 5).

Each question type has a *design* hierarchy of its own. In this section of the book, we focus mainly on questions relating to the health effects of *interventions* and *exposures*. These questions usually focus on how one *intervention* or *exposure* compares with another. A hierarchy of *designs* for studies addressing such issues is given in Box 1.4. The most sound *study design* in this context is one that randomly allocates (concealing the assignment code) *participants* to the alternative *interventions* of interest. This *design* serves to remove selection bias and, when conducted well, such studies rank at the top of the *study design* hierarchy for effectiveness evidence. Studies where the allocation of *participants* falls short of genuine randomization and allocation concealment have an inherent risk of bias, and in the evaluation of the strength of evidence, they are assigned a low level initially (Step 5). An inability to recognize valid *designs* can have serious implications for evidence-based practice. For example, relying on expert opinion when reviewing literature could mislead practice

Box 1.4 A simple hierarchy of *study designs* for questions about the effectiveness of healthcare interventions

Description of the *design*

Experimental study

A comparative study* in which the use of different interventions among participants is allocated by the researcher.

- **Randomized controlled trial (with concealed allocation)**
  Random allocation of participants to an intervention and a control (e.g. placebo or usual care) group, with follow-up to examine differences in outcomes between the two groups. Randomization (with concealment of allocation sequence from caregivers and participants) avoids bias because both known and unknown determinants of outcome, apart from the intervention, are usually equally distributed between the comparison groups.

- **Experimental study without randomization (sometimes called quasi-experimental or quasi-randomized or pseudo-randomized studies)**
  A study in which the allocation of participants to different interventions is managed by the researcher but the method of allocation falls short of genuine randomization, e.g. alternate or even-odd allocation. Such methods fail to conceal the allocation sequence from caregivers and participants.

Observational study with a control group

A comparative study* in which the use of different interventions among participants is not allocated by the researcher (it is merely observed).

- **Cohort study**
  Follow-up of participants who receive an intervention (that is not allocated by the researcher) to examine the difference in outcomes compared to a control group, e.g. participants receiving no care.
- **Case-control studies**
  Comparison of intervention rates between participant groups with the outcome (cases) and those without the outcome (controls).

Observational study without control groups

- **Cross-sectional study**
  Examination of the relationship between outcomes and other variables of interest (including interventions) as they exist in relevant participants at one particular time.
- **Before-and-after study**
  Comparison of outcomes in study participants before and after an intervention.
- **Case series**
  Description of a number of cases of an intervention and their outcomes.

Others

- Case reports which fail to establish a causal association due to the play of chance in individual cases
- Pathophysiological studies or bench research
- Expert opinion or consensus

* A comparative study assesses the effect of an intervention or exposure using comparison groups. See Box 1.1 for an example flow chart of such a study.

recommendations, e.g. erroneously withholding thrombolytic therapy in myocardial infarction, a field in which experts have lagged a decade behind strong evidence of the effect of this *intervention* on mortality (*JAMA* 1992; **268**: 240-8, doi:10.1001/jama.1992.03490020088036).

As indicated above, for many reviews, experimental studies will not exist (Case study 2) or they might be scarce (Case study 3). Hence, reviews may have to be conducted using studies of an inferior *design* or using studies with a mixture of *designs*. If our review has several *study designs*, it would be prudent to carefully plan study quality assessments (Step 3), stratify study synthesis by *design* and quality (Step 4) and interpret findings cautiously (Step 5). Reviewers who do not take a cautious approach to the *design* issue can easily produce erroneous conclusions. For example, initial recommendations that postmenopausal women use hormone replacement therapy to reduce cardiovascular risk came from observational studies with inconsistent results. Recognition of the limitations of the evidence would have tempered the recommendations, avoiding the need to reverse recommendations when randomized evidence showed that hormone replacement therapy fails to reduce cardiovascular risk and may even increase it (*Ann Intern Med* 2002; **137**: 273-84, doi: 10.7326/0003-4819-137-4-200208200-00012).

1.4 Narrow *versus* broad questions

Reviewers often face a tension between formulating questions with either a wide or a narrow focus. Practitioners think broadly about clinical topics before making a decision concerning a specific patient or problem. A typical systematic review, however, addresses a question about the comparison of a single *intervention* or *exposure versus* control. This approach can fail to take a broad perspective. The norm is that there are various treatment options for a condition. Considering the time and resources available, we may construct a narrowly focused question or we may go forward with a broad-based question for our review. The latter may involve conducting several narrowly focused reviews simultaneously within a review project. In a topic where we are likely to find several reviews already published, an umbrella review may collate their findings. In such a review, we choose systematic review as the *study design* for our question (Case study 1). Such umbrella reviews underpin clinical practice guidelines and serve as key knowledge sources for evidence-based practice (Case study 8).

An **umbrella review** is an evidence synthesis in the form of a review of systematic reviews on a topic. It may be a collation of all systematic reviews on a single narrowly focused question or it may bring together several different narrowly focused reviews to provide coverage of a broad question.

1.5 Review registration and protocol

It is important to demonstrate publicly that the question was formulated prospectively by registering the review in an online database like *Prospero* (crd.york.ac.uk/prospero, see Box 0.1) or OSF (Open Science Framework Registries, osf.io/registries). At this time, it is worth double-checking if reviews addressing your question don't already exist using the sources given in Box 0.1. Apart from helping to avoid waste of an effort in unnecessary duplication, it will also help in offering a justification for the review in the introduction section of the manuscript when submitting your paper for publication in a peer-reviewed journal. If there are no previous reviews or if the previous reviews have limitations in quality on critical appraisal, the justification for a new review will be clear for anyone to see (Case study 10).

Reviewers should also consider publishing their systematic review protocol in a peer-reviewed journal or uploading it on the prospective registration website. A review with only a few relevant studies will be completed too quickly for its protocol to be written up in line with a journal's instructions, submitted with its reporting requirements, peer-reviewed, revised, accepted and published. However, a large review project which may take several years to complete, e.g. a doctoral thesis based on systematic reviews, may benefit from formal publication of its protocol. When drafting a manuscript for publication of a review protocol, reporting guidelines available at the PRISMA platform may be required by the journal (prisma-statement.org/extensions/protocols.aspx). PRISMA provides a minimum set of items for transparently reporting systematic reviews, meta-analyses and their protocols. It focuses on reviews evaluating the effects of interventions using randomized trials and can be adapted for other systematic reviews that may evaluate other clinical areas such as test accuracy and disease prognosis.

Reporting guidelines are checklists for writing manuscripts. They provide a list of reporting items with a flow diagram to enhance the transparency of the manuscript (equator-network. org). Most journals require authors to submit a relevant systematic review reporting checklist (e.g. PRISMA, MOOSE, MARS, etc.). This assists peer-reviewers and editors in their assessment of compliance of the manuscript with good methodology and reporting standards.

1.6 Modification of questions during a review

It is important that review questions are formulated *a priori*, that is, before the review work is actually commenced. Otherwise, the review process may be unduly driven by presuming particular findings. To get the questions as correctly formulated as possible at the beginning, it may be worth involving experienced reviewers and practitioners in the process. This is just one of several reasons why it is considered unwise to prepare a review alone.

Questions will initially be developed without detailed knowledge of much of the relevant literature. Therefore, we should not be surprised if it becomes evident during the course of undertaking the review that some questions need to be modified in light of the accumulated research. The commandment 'thou shall pose questions for a review *a priori*' should not be applied too rigidly. We should allow exploration of unexpected issues into the review process; as a greater understanding of the problem is developed during the course of the review, it would be foolish not to do so. If the ongoing work identifies a need for answering questions which had not been foreseen, it would be quite reasonable to raise new questions or modify existing questions. Such modifications are justifiable if they are based on the realization of alternative ways of defining the *participants, interventions, outcomes* or *study designs*, which were not considered earlier.

Revision of questions will inevitably have some implications for the review work. The protocol would have to be revised. Literature searches (Step 2), which are usually conducted before questions are refined, may also need refinement and they might have to be run again in the light of the changes to the questions. Study selection criteria will have to be altered. For example, in the review of the safety of water fluoridation in Case study 2, the original questions were modified in the light of information gathered about the extent and range of quality of available evidence during the initial part of the review. This led to changes in study selection criteria, which are provided in detail in the published report of the review (york.ac.uk/inst/crd/fluorid.htm). Reviewers should not be economical with the truth about question formulation and refinement at the time of writing up manuscripts for publication. For transparency, it is essential to be explicit about the modifications and indicate which questions were posed *a priori* and which were generated during the review work. Some journals may require a transparency declaration at the time of submission of their systematic review manuscript asking authors to affirm that any changes from the planned review have been explained. This is aided by prospective registration before conducting the review.

Writing tips for systematic review authors

- **Publication type:** Most journals that publish systematic reviews have specific instructions for this article type. Read the instructions for authors concerning this article type in the chosen journal. Some journals exclusively publish review articles. Beware, many journals routinely carry out plagiarism checks. In addition to the journal's instructions, follow the relevant reporting guidelines or comply with as many of the PRISMA reporting items as applicable. Most journals require authors to submit a reporting checklist along with the manuscript.
- **Title:** Definitely state that your manuscript is about a systematic review. Keep title length within the character limit prescribed by the journal. Include as many components of the review question in the title as possible. Write the design subheading, stating whether it is a systematic review with or without a meta-analysis or an umbrella review or another review type. Ensure that the title in the manuscript matches the prospectively registered title. Ensure that the

IMRaD is an acronym that refers to the section headings used in writing the main manuscript text, i.e. I-Introduction, M-Methods, R-Results, a-and D-Discussion, of a systematic review paper for submission to a peer-reviewed journal. See Case study 10 for tips, tricks and unwritten rules for convincing journal editors and peer-reviewers to publish your article.

title, the objective statement in the abstract and the last paragraph of the introduction all sing from the same hymn sheet with respect to the review question.

- **Abstract:** Write the abstract first! Keep returning to it to revise and improve it as the rest of the main text is drafted. Use a structured format. Stay within the permitted word limits. If your chosen journal wants an unstructured abstract, the subheadings can be removed and the sentences merged into a paragraph after the structured abstract has been finalized. Write the objective statement covering all the components of the review question. Provide the prospective registration details. Abbreviations should be accompanied by full descriptions. The abstract should be able to stand alone without the need to refer to the main text to understand its contents.
- **Introduction:** Cover both the objective and the design from the abstract in the last paragraph of the introduction describing the review question.
- **Methods:** Provide the prospective registration details again. If a protocol has been published, refer to it. Describe any protocol modification transparently. In addition to reporting any modification to the planned review in the methods section, give a transparency declaration in the cover letter even if not formally required by the journal. Some journals may require you to provide the protocol as supplementary material to accompany the manuscript. Patient and public involvement, required as an obligatory part of the manuscript by many journals, can be included in a subsection describing, for example, how lay input was sought in the choice of *outcomes* when framing the review question. Refer to a core *outcomes* set if one was used in question formulation.
- **Discussion:** Comment on the role played by the patient and public involvement in framing the question, particularly focusing on determining the importance of the outcomes. If the review covers a narrowly focused question, provide a discussion about what its findings mean compared to the evidence available concerning other questions in the topic broadly.

Summary of Step 1: Framing questions for a review

Key points about appraising review articles

- Examine the abstract and the methods to see if the review is based on predefined questions. Look for information concerning prospective registration.
- Examine the methods and other sections to check if questions were modified during the review process.
- Can we be sure that the questions have not been unduly influenced by the knowledge of the results of the studies?

Key points about conducting reviews

- The problems to be addressed by the review should be specified in the form of clear, unambiguous questions before beginning the review work.
- Questions should be structured, e.g. in terms of *participants, interventions, outcomes* and *study designs* relevant to the issues being addressed in the review.
- Characteristics of the *participants*, differences in *interventions*, variation in *outcomes* and variety in *study designs* may influence the results of a review. The impact of these factors should be carefully considered at this stage.
- Prospectively and publicly register the review in a database like *Prospero* or OSF Registries.
- Consider publishing a systematic protocol in a peer-reviewed journal or uploading the protocol on the prospective registration website.
- Once the review questions have been set, modifications to the protocol should only be allowed after careful consideration. Sometimes, alternative ways of defining the *participants, interventions, outcomes* or *study designs* become apparent after commencing the review. In this situation, it would be reasonable to alter the original questions, but these modifications should not be driven by the knowledge of the results of the studies.

Step 2: *Identifying relevant literature*

Step 1
Framing questions
↓
Step 2
Identifying relevant literature
↓
Step 3
Assessing the quality of the literature
↓
Step 4
Summarizing the evidence
↓
Step 5
Interpreting the findings

Being thorough when identifying the relevant literature is crucial for a systematic review. It is driven by the desire to capture as many relevant studies as possible. In published reviews, literature searches are often summarized too simplistically to allow others to replicate them. A good search can vary between simple and relatively complex, depending on the review topic. Not all searches are beyond the reach of novice reviewers.

A comprehensive literature search includes multistage and iterative processes. First, we will need to generate lists of citations from relevant resources (e.g. electronic bibliographic databases, reference lists of known primary and review articles and relevant journals). Second, we will need to screen these citations for relevance to our review questions with a view to obtaining the full manuscripts of all potentially relevant studies. Third, we will need to sift through these manuscripts to make the final inclusion/exclusion decisions based on explicit study selection criteria. Some of the studies will provide reference lists from which we will find more potentially relevant citations, and the cycle of obtaining manuscripts and examining them for relevance will go one more round. These processes will eventually lead to a set of studies on which the review will be based. In the manuscript of our review, a flow chart of the study identification process will be required (Box 2.1). The basic principles behind the identification of relevant literature covering various aspects of this flow chart are covered in this Step.

2.1 Generating a list of potentially relevant citations

Both the precision and the validity of the findings of reviews are directly related to the comprehensiveness of the literature identification processes. The aim of the initial searches is to generate as comprehensive a list of citations as possible to address the questions being posed in the review. Thus, the search strategy (search terms and the resources to be searched) will depend on the components of the questions. If we have formulated the questions well, we have already made a head start. In practical terms, developing a search strategy may take several iterations, so we should be prepared for the hard work. However, using a systematic approach (similar to the one outlined below) can quickly lead us to a reasonably effective strategy.

The steps involved in electronically generating lists of potentially relevant citations include a selection of relevant databases, formulation of an appropriate combination of search terms and retrieval of citations from the searches. Searches undertaken at the beginning of the review may have to be updated at a later date depending on the length of time taken to complete the review.

Precision of effect in a review refers to its uncertainty. Poor searches may contribute to uncertainty by identifying only a fraction of the available studies, which leads to wide confidence intervals around the summary effects. **Imprecision** refers to uncertainty arising due to play of chance, but not due to **bias**.

Validity of a review refers to the methods used to minimize **bias**. **Bias** will either exaggerate or underestimate the 'true' effect being sought in a review. Poor searches contribute to **bias** as they may preferentially identify studies with particularly positive or particularly negative effects.

DOI: 10.1201/9781003220039-3

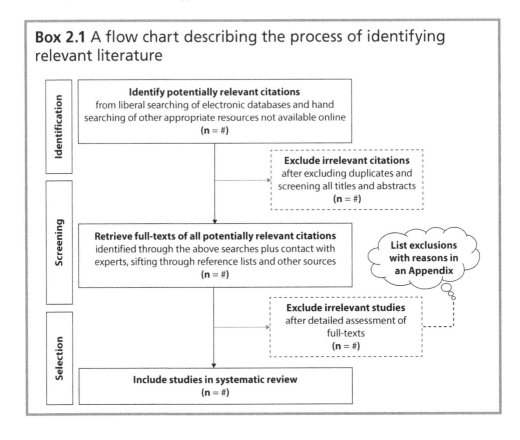

Box 2.1 A flow chart describing the process of identifying relevant literature

Identification

Identify potentially relevant citations
from liberal searching of electronic databases and hand searching of other appropriate resources not available online
(n = #)

Exclude irrelevant citations
after excluding duplicates and screening all titles and abstracts
(n = #)

Screening

Retrieve full-texts of all potentially relevant citations
identified through the above searches plus contact with experts, sifting through reference lists and other sources
(n = #)

List exclusions with reasons in an Appendix

Exclude irrelevant studies
after detailed assessment of full-texts
(n = #)

Selection

Include studies in systematic review
(n = #)

2.1.1 Selection of relevant databases to search

There exists no such database that covers all publications from all healthcare journals. Serious reviewers usually search many databases. How should we decide about database coverage? This depends very much on the topic of the review. Why not compare and contrast the types of databases searched in Case study 2 (Box C2.1) with those searched in Case study 3 (Box C3.1): the differences are mainly due to differences in the nature of the review topics. There are many useful databases and we may wish to ask our local librarian or consult one of the guides to databases. Some of the commonly used databases are given in Box 2.2.

Most reviews would include searches in general databases such as Medline and Embase, which cover many of the same journals. Medline is produced by the US National Library of Medicine and has a North American emphasis. Embase has a greater European emphasis in terms of the journals it covers and has a high pharmacological content. Local medical libraries or professional bodies may provide free access to both Medline and Embase. To complicate matters for novice reviewers, there are a number of different online interfaces for electronic databases, e.g. Medline is available

---

Box 2.2 Important databases of research in healthcare

Selected general databases

- **Medline** (available freely via PubMed at ncbi.nlm.nih.gov/PubMed)
- Bibliographic records (with and without abstracts) or citations from 1966 onwards. Related articles is a feature useful for systematic reviews.
- **Embase** (embase.com)
- Records of biomedical literature from 1947 onwards.
- **Web of Science** (webofscience.com)
- Established as a Science Citation Index in 1964, it contains citations from over 9000 journals. Citation search is a feature useful for systematic reviews.
- **Google Scholar** (scholar.google.com)
- Established in 2004, Scholar is a massive online platform that keeps up with new research and non-conventional or grey literature. Cross references with other sources is a feature useful for systematic reviews.

Selected databases with a specific focus

- **PsycInfo** (psycinfo.apa.org)
- Records of literature on psychology, behavioural and social sciences from 1967.
- **Central** (cochranelibrary.com/central)
- The Cochrane Central Register of Controlled Trials contains records of clinical trials in healthcare identified from some of the general databases above as well as trial registries.
- **Cinahl** (cinahl.com)
- The Cumulative Index to Nursing and Allied Health Literature.
- **Midirs** (midirs.org)
- A broad reference resource available to obstetricians, midwives and consumers.
- **Research Registers** (for research in progress, e.g. isrctn.com)
- The ISRCTN registry is freely accessible and searchable.

See Boxes C2.1, C3.2, C5.1 and C6.1 for some other databases searched in the Case studies.

---

via PubMed as well as Ovid. The mode of searching in commercial platforms like Ovid is flexible and user-friendly, but they are more costly than the PubMed interface to Medline, which is freely available on the Internet. The PubMed interface has an additional searching feature via its 'Related Articles' function, which allows the capture of additional citations on the basis of their similarity to known relevant citations.

As research is nowadays published and accessed readily on the Internet, it is worth looking at how the Worldwide Web can also be used to supplement formal electronic database searches for completed studies. It can help identify researchers and manufacturers as well as ongoing studies. Given the enormity of the Web, any serious attempt to search it would be a major undertaking, with tens of thousands of web pages to browse. A structured approach would have to be developed, e.g. using meta-search engines that aggregate searches from various search engines like Dogpile – dogpile.com and search engines with a healthcare focus, e.g. Turning Research Into Practice – tripdatabase.com (see Case study 8), EvidenceAlerts – evidencealerts.com, etc., but this approach is tailored to support evidence-based clinical decisions, not systematic reviews.

2.1.2 Search term combination for electronic database searches

In simple terms, building a suitable combination of search terms involves combining free text words and controlled terms (MeSH or MeSH-like terms) which represent the various components of the review question.

We should begin by examining the *participants, interventions* or *exposures, outcomes* and *study designs* relevant to our review, as shown in Box 2.3. For each one of these components, we will need to compile a list of words that authors might have used in their studies. We may identify a range of synonyms with spelling variations by examining the relevant studies we already know of. These will provide the free text words for our search. We will also need to compile a list of controlled terms that database indexers might have used when recording the citations. There are many ways to identify relevant MeSH or MeSH-like terms. For example, we may look at the key words suggested for indexing in known relevant studies (frequently found at the end of the abstract) and check how they are actually indexed in the databases we want to search. We need to keep in mind that indexers don't always follow authors' suggestions. Each database has its own thesaurus or index structure and we may want to refer to this for additional MeSH terms. This task is made easier in databases that offer the opportunity to map free text words we have selected to MeSH in their index lists. However, when we select our search terms, we must ensure that an adequate number of free text words and controlled terms are included to represent each component of the question. This will enhance the sensitivity of our search, increasing our ability to capture a large proportion of the relevant studies.

The next stage is to combine the words and terms we have selected to capture the various components of the question. This is achieved by Boolean logic which commonly uses the operators AND, OR and NOT to create sets of citations from the search terms. For example, combining *coke* OR *cola* will retrieve all citations where either one or both of these terms are found. On the other hand, combining *coke* AND *cola* will only retrieve citations where both of these terms are found. Combining *coke* NOT *cola* will retrieve citations that contain the term *coke* only, thereby excluding all citations with the term *cola*. Needless to say, NOT should be used with great caution. In general, one would use OR to combine all the words and terms capturing a component of the question. This will give a large citation set for each component that we searched for. We can now combine these with AND to produce a set which contains citations relevant to all the various components of the question.

MeSH or medical subject headings are controlled terms used in the Medline database to index citations. Other bibliographic databases use MeSH-like terms.

Sensitivity of a search is the proportion of relevant studies identified by a search strategy expressed as a percentage of all relevant studies on a given topic. It is a measure of the comprehensiveness of a search method. *Do not confuse it with a sensitivity of a test.*

Boolean logic refers to the logical relationship among search terms.

Boolean operators AND, OR and NOT are used during literature searches to include or exclude certain citations from electronic databases. An example of their use in PubMed is shown below:

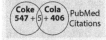

Coke = **552**
Cola = **411**
Coke **AND** Cola = **5**
Coke **OR** Cola = **958**
Coke **NOT** Cola = **547**

Box 2.3 How to develop a search term combination for searching electronic bibliographic databases

An example of a search term combination for Ovid Medline database

Free-form question: In women undergoing surgical termination of pregnancy, does antibiotic prophylaxis reduce the risk of post-operative infection?

Structured question (not all components may be needed for searching)

• The participants	Pregnant women undergoing surgical abortion
• The interventions	• Antibiotics used as prophylaxis
	• Comparator: Placebo or no intervention (not used in search term combination)
• The outcome	Post-operative infection
• The study design	Experimental studies (not used in search term combination)

Question components and relevant search terms	Type of terms		Boolean operator
	Free	MeSH	
The participants: Pregnant women undergoing surgical abortion			
1 (terminat$ adj3 pregnan$).tw	x		
2 (unwant$ adj3 pregnan$).tw	x		
3 abortion$.tw	x		OR (captures *participants*)
4 exp abortion induced/		x	
5 exp pregnancy unwanted/		x	
6 or/1–5			
The interventions: Antibiotics used as prophylaxis			
7 exp infection control/		x	
8 exp anti-infective agents/		x	
9 exp antibiotics/		x	
10 antibiotic$.tw	x		OR (captures *interventions*)
11 (antibiotic adj3 prophyla$).tw	x		
12 (antimicrobial$ or anti-microbial$).tw	x		
13 or/7–12			
The outcome: Post-operative infection			
14 exp bacterial infections/		x	
15 exp postoperative complications/		x	
16 sepsis/		x	
17 exp abortion septic/		x	
18 exp endometritis/		x	
19 exp adnexitis/		x	
20 (postoperative adj3 (infect$ or contaminat$ or complicat$ or pyrexi$)).tw	x		OR (captures *outcome*)
21 (sepsis or septic).tw	x		

Question components and relevant search terms	Type of terms		Boolean operator
	Free	MeSH	
22 (bacteria$ adj3 (contaminat$ or infect$)).tw	x		
23 (post-abort$ adj3 (infect$ or complicat$ or contaminat$)).tw	x		
24 endometritis.tw	x		
25 pelvic inflammatory disease.tw	x		
26 (septic adj3 abort$).tw	x		
27 or/14–26			
28 and/6,13,27			AND (combines all components)

Commands and symbols for Ovid Medline

$ Truncation, e.g. pregnan$, will pick up pregnant, pregnancy and pregnancies adj Proximity and adjacency searching, e.g. terminat$ adj pregnan$ means that these terms appear next to each other, terminat$ adj3 pregnan$ means that there may be three other words in between them

.tw   Textword search, e.g. abortion$.tw, will search for text words in title or abstract

/   Medical subject heading (MeSH) search, e.g. abortion induced/, will search for MeSH in indexing terms

adj(n) Proximity searches for terms a specified number (n) spaces away from each other, e.g. septic adj3 abort$ will search for abortion within 3 spaces of septic. If (n) is not specified, only a single space is used.

Exp   Explodes the MeSH, e.g. exp abortion induced/will search for this MeSH as well as the lower order MeSH terms included under the MeSH abortion induced in tree structure, such as abortion eugenic, abortion legal, abortion therapeutic, pregnancy reduction multifetal

See related selection criteria in Box 2.4.

Box 2.3 only shows the search term combinations for the Medline database. Any search term combinations developed for Medline would need to be adapted to the peculiarities of each of the other databases to be searched. This may require professional support. It can be guaranteed that this will not be easy, particularly because different databases use different terms and index structures. But we should not lose sight of our objective, which is to produce a valid answer to the questions raised for the review. There is substantial evidence that limiting the search to only a few databases tends to bias the review. Limitations by language and date do the same. The more broad based our search, the more likely it is that our review will produce a precise and valid answer.

2.1.3 Searching for study designs

One important component of the review question is the *study design*, which can be used to improve our search strategy. For example, to identify published and unpublished clinical trials, we may search specialist collections such as the Cochrane Central Register of Controlled Trials

(Central) and research registers of ongoing trials (clinicaltrials.gov). These are usually the first databases to be searched in reviews of randomized studies. However, for other *study designs*, such collections are rare.

General databases have subject indexing for some study designs, but this alone may not be adequate for searching. Therefore, search term combinations which capture studies of a particular design (also known as search filters) have been developed by information specialists. It is tempting to search general databases using such *design* filters, e.g. in PubMed searches can be restricted to randomized trials. Some filters are designed to perform quick searches to support day-to-day evidence-based practice. They will make our search more precise, but inevitably this will be at the expense of sensitivity. This means that a high proportion of citations retrieved by filtered searches will be relevant, but many relevant citations will be missed because they are not indexed in a way that the filter can pick up. This is a major drawback because systematic reviews should be based on searches that are as thorough as possible. There is one exception – for reviews of randomized trials where indexing of *design*-related terms is more reasonable, carefully adapted versions of existing filters for therapy questions may be used (Case study 3). Case study 5 demonstrates the use of a qualitative research design filter (Box C5.1).

Precision of a search or its specificity is the proportion of relevant studies identified by a search strategy. This is expressed as a percentage of all studies (relevant and irrelevant) identified by that strategy. It is a measure of the ability of a search to exclude irrelevant studies. Do not confuse with the precision of effect.

Study design filter employs a search term combination to capture citations of studies of a particular *design*.

2.1.4 Reference lists and other sources (e.g. grey literature, conference proceedings)

Inaccurate or incomplete indexing of articles and journals in electronic bibliographic databases requires the examination of other sources of citations. Reference lists from identified studies and related reviews provide a rich source of potentially relevant citations and these can usually be downloaded for examination alongside the database searches. Index Medicus and Excerpta Medica used to be manually searched if it was desirable to identify studies prior to the start dates of the electronic databases (as in Case study 2). The latest issues of the key journals also used to be searched to identify the most recent studies which were yet to be included in the electronic databases or cited by others. Nowadays citations and preprints appear online before the papers are published formally.

Many studies published in technical reports, discussion papers or other formats are not included in major databases and journals, but they can usually be captured by online searches. The libraries of specialist research organizations and professional societies may provide another useful source of this grey literature. Dissertations and theses can also be routes to obtaining otherwise unpublished research and these are recorded in databases such as Dissertation Abstracts, oatd.org (Open access theses and dissertations), Cinahl (Cumulative Index to Nursing and Allied Health Literature), etc. Conference proceedings, included in Google

Scholar, can provide information on research in progress as well as completed research. Gone are the days when one had to visit large research libraries to search manually for information.

2.1.5 Identifying ongoing research

The most unbiased study retrieval can only be guaranteed in those areas where prospective comprehensive research registers are maintained. These research registers may provide information on planned, ongoing or completed studies. Box 2.2 shows an electronic resource to search for ongoing studies. Many pharmaceutical companies hold their study results in private databases, which may be released on request.

Bias in study retrieval will either exaggerate or underestimate the 'true' effect being sought in a review. Poor searches contribute to **bias** as they may preferentially identify studies with particularly positive or particularly negative effects.

2.1.6 Seeking professional input

After reading through this section, you might feel that literature identification is beyond your current searching skills and you will need professional input. Many professional reviewers receive support from information specialists to carry out their searches. Your local librarian may be able to help – they might be able to direct you to an information service that conducts systematic literature searches. Registering your review with a relevant Review Group of the Cochrane Collaboration might allow you access to professional searches. Many of the Review Groups have developed comprehensive search strategies for their topics and maintain specialized registers.

2.2 Citation retrieval and management

In order to effectively manage the process of literature identification, citations obtained from the searches will have to be imported into a computer program for reference management (e.g. Reference Manager, EndNote, Mendeley, Zotero). The construction of a master citation database for a review will involve collating all the citations from various sources. Built-in functions of the citation management software allow exact and inexact duplicates (where titles, authors or journal names of the same articles are cited or stated in different manners) to be easily detected and removed. Additional functions of the software can add labels or tags to the citations, by the creation of user defined fields, allowing for enhanced sorting and documentation of the selection process. Searches of some of the sources (e.g. Central) may not be importable directly into the master citation database. Citations from these sources will have to be scrutinized and managed by importing them individually into reference management files and folders. In addition, searches of non-electronic sources (e.g. reference lists of known articles not available online) may have to be managed manually. Eventually, many citations will have to be individually entered into the master

The **Cochrane Collaboration** is an international collaboration that aims to help with informed decision-making on healthcare by preparing, maintaining and ensuring accessibility of systematic reviews of interventions (cochrane.org).

citation database of the review. The citation manager should also plug in into the word processing program to facilitate the writing of the manuscript for publication.

2.3 Selecting relevant studies

The aim of the study selection process is to use the citation lists to identify those articles that definitely address the questions being posed in the review. This is part of the multistage process described in Box 2.1. The process consists of defining the study selection criteria, screening the citations to obtain the full reports of all studies that are likely to meet the selection criteria and sifting through these manuscripts to make the final inclusion/exclusion decisions.

2.3.1 Study selection criteria

These should follow on logically from the review question. Box 2.4 shows example sets of selection criteria defined in terms of the *participants*, *interventions* or *exposures*, *outcome* and *study designs* of interest. Ultimately, only studies that meet all of the inclusion criteria (and none of the exclusion criteria) will be included in the review. To avoid bias in the selection process, the criteria (both inclusion and exclusion) should be defined *a priori*.

When defining selection criteria, we should ask ourselves:

- Is it sensible to group various *participants* together?
- Is it sensible to combine various *interventions* together?
- What *outcomes* are clinically relevant?
- What *study designs* should be included/excluded?

Often reviewers are led by what is likely to be reported rather than by what is clinically important, but it is preferable to select studies with clinical importance rather than surrogate *outcomes* (Step 1). The decision taken about study selection, whatever it is, will have consequences for the rest of the review. It is up to us as the reviewers to decide on how broad or narrow the selection criteria should be. Criteria that are too broadly defined may make it difficult to synthesize studies; criteria that are too narrowly defined may reduce the applicability of the findings of our review. A balanced approach can enhance the applicability of our findings. For example, using liberal inclusion criteria concerning the *participants* may allow investigation of questions concerning the variation in effects among different *participant* subgroups (see Box 4.5).

Ideally, studies of the most robust *design* should be included. However, practically, the criteria concerning *study design* may be influenced by knowing the type and amount of available literature to some extent after initiating the review. If the selection criteria are modified in the light of the information gathered from the initial searches, the modifications should be justified and explicitly reported. When studies of

Selecting relevant studies
- Develop selection criteria based on the structured question
- Screen downloaded searches for potentially relevant citations
- Obtain full-texts or pdf files of papers and select those relevant
- Exclude citations and full-texts that have been retracted
- Do not use language or date restrictions
- Undertake assessments in duplicate resolving disagreements through discussion or arbitration

Box 2.4 Some examples of study selection criteria

Free-form question: In women undergoing surgical termination of pregnancy, does antibiotic prophylaxis reduce the risk of post-operative infection? (*see the structured question in Box 2.3*)

Question component	Inclusion criteria	Exclusion criteria
● The participants	Pregnant women undergoing surgical abortion	Other operations
● The interventions	Antibiotics compared to placebo or no prophylaxis; comparison of different antibiotics	Lack of comparison
● The outcome	Post-operative infection confirmed by appropriate microbiological techniques	Infection not confirmed
● The study design	Experimental studies	Observational studies

Free-form question: Is it safe to provide population-wide drinking water fluoridation to prevent caries?

Question component	Inclusion criteria	Exclusion criteria
● The participants	People receiving drinking water sourced through a public water supply	Unsourced water supply
● The interventions	Fluoridation of drinking water, naturally occurring or artificially added, compared to non-fluoridated water	Lack of comparison
● The outcome	Cancer, bone fractures and fluorosis	Other outcomes
● The study design	– Experimental studies – Observational studies (cohort, case-control, cross-sectional, and before-and-after)	– Case series – Case reports

See Case study 2 for a related review.

Free-form question: Which of the many available antimicrobial products improve healing in patients with chronic wounds? (*see the structured question in Box 1.3*)

Question component	Inclusion criteria	Exclusion criteria
● The participants	Adults with chronic wounds	Other wounds
● The interventions	Systemic and topical antimicrobial preparations compared to placebo or no antimicrobial; comparison of different antibiotics	Lack of comparison
● The outcome	Wound healing	Wound healing not assessed

Question component	Inclusion criteria	Exclusion criteria
• The study design	– Randomized controlled trials – Experimental studies without randomization – Cohort studies with concurrent controls	– Studies with historical controls – Case-control studies

See Case study 3 for a related review.
See Box 1.4 *for a brief description of various study designs.*

robust *designs* have not been carried out (Case study 2) or if they are scarce (Case study 3), the inclusion criterion specifying the *study design* may have to consider studies of methodologically poorer quality. This approach may be used in reviews where the goal is to summarize the currently available evidence for decision-making, as in Case studies 2, 3 and 6. If a review has several *study designs*, this will have implications on study quality assessments (Step 3), study synthesis (Step 4) and interpretation of findings (which should be cautious) based mainly on methodologically superior studies (Step 5).

2.3.2 Screening of citations

Initially, the selection criteria should be applied liberally to the citation lists generated from searching relevant literature sources. Citations often contain only limited information, so any titles (and abstracts) which seem potentially relevant should provisionally be included for consideration on the basis of the full-text articles. However, many citations will clearly be irrelevant and these can be excluded at this stage. This task can be quite subjective, so it is advisable that two reviewers should carry out citation screening independently and the full manuscripts of all citations considered relevant by any of the reviewers should be obtained. The yield of this process will vary from one review to another. Applying a little foresight, keeping in mind the publication of your review in due course, capture citations to systematic reviews on your topic and set them aside. They will prove useful for writing the introduction and discussion sections of your review article.

2.3.3 Obtaining full-texts of manuscripts

In the past, one visited the library to find out the lists and dates of journals available locally. Nowadays, the Internet offers freely available journals (freemedicaljournals.com) and papers for download electronically. Your institution or library may also subscribe to electronic journals not freely available. In this way, many recent publications may be quickly obtained. The next Step will be to obtain articles not available through our library or on the Internet. This could be time-consuming and help from the local librarian or a librarian at a professional body will be invaluable.

On occasion, it may be necessary to write to the authors directly to obtain the papers. The professional network for scientists and researchers such as ResearchGate (researchgate.net) offers access to authors and papers.

2.3.4 Study selection

The final inclusion/exclusion decisions should be made after examining the full-texts of all the potentially relevant citations. We should carefully assess the information contained in these to see whether the criteria have been met or not. Many of the doubtful citations initially included may be confidently excluded at this stage. It will be useful to construct a list of excluded studies at this point, detailing the reason for each exclusion. This will not take much time and providing this list as part of our review increases the quality of our manuscript for publication. With the publication of papers on the Internet, there are fewer restrictions on space as details of searches and selection typically not included in the main text of the manuscript can be provided as supplements or appendices to go along with the published paper.

Two independent reviewers should undertake assessments of citations and full-texts of articles for selection because even when explicit inclusion criteria are prespecified, the decisions concerning inclusion/exclusion can be relatively subjective. For example, when applying the *study design* criteria for selection, reviewers may disagree about including or excluding a study due to unclear or erroneous reporting in the paper. For observational studies, it is well known that the assignment of case-control *design* by authors and its assessment by peer-reviewers is frequently erroneous, so reviewers cannot just accept what is reported in published articles without deliberation. The selection criteria can be initially piloted in a subset of studies where duplicate assessments allow reviewers to assess whether they can be applied in a consistent fashion. If the agreement between the reviewers is poor in the pilot phase, revision of the selection criteria may be required. Once these issues have been clarified, any subsequent disagreements are usually simple oversights, which are easily resolved by consensus. Arbitration by a third reviewer may be required when consensus cannot be reached. The degree of agreement between reviewers should be calculated in order to assess the reliability of the selection process. Beware of reviews which have only one or two authors; it is likely that errors will have been made in selecting studies.

2.3.5 Selecting studies with duplicate publication

Reviewers often encounter multiple publications of the same study. Prior to the publication of results, there may be reports of registrations and protocols. Sometimes there will be an exact duplication of results, but at other times there might be serial publications with the more recent papers reporting increasing numbers of participants or lengths of follow-up. Inclusion of duplicated data would inevitably add spurious precision, but it will also bias the data synthesis in the review, particularly because studies with more positive results are more likely to be duplicated. However, the examination of multiple reports of the same study may provide useful information about its quality and other characteristics not captured by a single report. Therefore, all such reports should be examined. However, the data should only be counted once using the largest, most complete report with the longest follow-up.

2.4 Publication and related biases

Identification of all the relevant studies depends on their accessibility. Some studies may be less accessible due to a lack of statistical significance in their results, the type and language of their reports, the timing of their publication and their indexing in databases, amongst other reasons.

> **Publication bias** is said to arise when the likelihood of publication of studies and thus their accessibility to reviewers is related to the significance of their results regardless of their quality.

Studies in which *interventions* are not found to be effective are less likely to be published or they are published in less accessible formats. Publication bias may also involve studies that report certain positive effects that go against prevailing beliefs. Systematic reviews that fail to identify such studies will inevitably exaggerate or underestimate the effect of an *intervention* and this is when publication bias arises. Thus, the use of a systematic approach to track down less accessible studies is crucial for avoiding bias in systematic reviews. Hopefully, with the prospective registration of primary studies, there will be less concern about overlooking studies. It is necessary to search hard to protect reviews against publication bias. In Step 4, we see how the risk of publication and related biases can be investigated in a review using a funnel plot analysis (Box 4.9).

2.4.1 Searching multiple databases

There is evidence that limiting the search to only a few databases tends to bias the review. Using the databases listed in Box 2.2, we need to cast as wide a net as possible to capture as many citations as possible. When searching randomized trials, it is recommended not just to search Central alone; at least Medline and Embase should also be searched alongside. Case studies 2 and 3 demonstrate the great lengths serious reviewers can go to when searching for citations. Similarly, if our review is to be taken seriously, we will have to search multiple (overlapping) sources of citations.

2.4.2 Language restrictions in study selection

There is no good reason for excluding articles published in languages that we cannot read or understand. There is increasing evidence that studies with positive findings are more likely to be published in English language journals. Studies with negative findings from non-English speaking countries may be published in local language journals. Therefore, positive studies are more likely to be accessed if searches are limited to the English language, thereby introducing bias. In addition, language restrictions may decrease the precision of the summary effect in our meta-analysis. For these reasons, it is necessary to work collaboratively. Accessing translation and interpretation facilities can be expensive. If our review is registered with a relevant Cochrane Review Group, there might be help available for dealing with multiple languages. Nowadays we may tackle this issue by joining various social media groups through which reviewers engage worldwide. This way we can easily ask researchers with competence in languages other than our own to extract the necessary data for us when we encounter papers in other languages. Translation software can quickly convert the language of a foreign language paper into our native language, but these tend not to have high fidelity in science literature translation as technical language is often not the same as spoken language.

2.4.3 Automation of literature searches

There is good reason to believe that the future developments in the computer sciences will help reviewers. Artificial intelligence can be deployed to automate systematic reviews, particularly Step 2. Information retrieval software can efficiently perform literature searches to help perform rapid reviews and to update living systematic reviews and guidelines. Such software uses computer science techniques such as machine learning, natural language processing and data mining amongst others. Once fully developed, they will have the potential to complement and substitute reviewer effort. This area is very much in its infancy at the time of writing our book as current systematic reviews have not frequently deployed artificial intelligence.

Rapid reviews are systematic reviews undertaken with urgency to synthesize evidence. **Living systematic reviews** and **living guidelines** are continually updated so as to keep the evidence synthesis up to date. Artificial intelligence has the potential to help achieve these ideals.

Writing tips for systematic review authors

- Use a suitable reference management software that plugs into the word processing software for citing literature in the main text and generating a bibliography while writing the manuscript, and also supports literature search and selection in Step 2. Beware that some journals may not accept reviews with searches completed more than 6 months prior to submission. The initial searches may have to be updated during a long review project just before finalizing the manuscript for submission. Search updates may also be required if the peer review takes too long.
- **Abstract:** Provide the resources searched with dates, making clear if any language or time restrictions were applied, and give selection criteria that explicitly match the review question.

- **Introduction:** When screening citations for relevant studies, capture and set aside all previous systematic review citations on your topic. They provide a handy source of references for drafting a strong background and justification in the paper. This is one of the keys to avoiding rejection immediately following submission (Box C10.1). Editors can strike you out even without a peer review if the justification for undertaking your review is weak.
- **Methods:** In the literature search and selection subsection, provide the resources searched with dates, making clear if any time or language restrictions were applied. Provide information about the search term combination deployed in at least one publicly available database. Ensure it maps to the review question. Details of adaptations of the search term combination in other databases can be included as supplementary material, usually Appendix 1. Describe study selection criteria, ensuring they are integrally linked to the review question. Specify study design-related selection criteria. In the selection process, cover how assessments to select studies were undertaken in duplicate and what was done to resolve disagreements amongst reviewers through discussion or arbitration. If agreement statistics are computed, these are typically described under the statistical analysis subsection.
- **Results:** Following the relevant reporting guideline, include in the subsection concerning literature search and selection the flow chart of study selection, usually Figure 1. Reference lists of excluded studies can be provided with reasons as supplementary material. Any agreement statistics computed concerning searches are typically reported at the end of the paragraph describing the study selection. Results of funnel plot analyses undertaken to explore the risk of publication and related biases are typically reported at the end of the results section.
- **Flow chart:** Give it a detailed title for it to stand alone. Simply stating 'Figure 1: Study selection flow chart' is insufficient. Clarify which review the flow chart pertains to including elements of the review question, e.g. 'Figure 1: Flow chart of study selection in the systematic review of antibiotic prophylaxis for surgical pregnancy termination'. Include relevant appendices within the boxes of the flow chart avoiding the need to refer to the text.
- **Discussion:** In the strength and weaknesses subsection, cover how the literature search and selection potentially impacted on precision and validity of the main findings of the review. The extent to which the literature was geographically spread may also have implications for the generalizability of the findings of the review. When comparing your findings with previous reviews, use the citations to systematic reviews about your topic which you captured during the screening of citations for relevant studies.

IMRaD is an acronym that refers to the section headings used in writing the main manuscript text, i.e. I-Introduction, M-Methods, R-Results, a-and, D-Discussion, of a systematic review paper for submission to a peer-reviewed journal. See Case study 10 for tips, tricks and unwritten rules for convincing journal editors and peer-reviewers to publish your article.

Summary of Step 2: Identifying relevant literature

Key points about appraising review articles

- Examine the abstract and the methods section to see if the searches appear to be comprehensive:
  - Check if search term combinations follow from the question.
  - List the resources (e.g. databases) searched to identify primary studies.
  - Have any relevant resources been left out?
  - Were any restrictions applied by dates, language, etc.?
- Were the selection criteria set *a priori*? How reliably were they applied?
- Have analyses been conducted to examine for the risk of publication and related biases? (see Step 4)
- How likely is it that relevant studies might have been missed? And what is the potential impact on the conclusions of the review?

Key points about conducting reviews

- The search for studies should be extensive and the selection process should minimize bias.
- The search term combination should follow from the question with the proper translation of structured question components into subject headings and free text terms.
- The search term combination should be designed to cast a wide net for capturing as many potentially relevant citations as possible. Boolean and proximity operators should be carefully applied to minimize the risk of unintentional exclusions. The choice of any *study design* filters should be carefully mapped to the question.
- Multiple resources should be searched. Searches undertaken at the beginning may have to be updated towards the end of the review, depending on the length of time taken to review.
- A systematic approach to citation management should be used to manage the review efficiently.
- Study selection criteria should flow directly from the review questions; they should be set *a priori* and should be piloted to check that they can be reliably applied.
- When sifting through the citations, selection criteria should be applied liberally to retrieve full-text manuscripts of all potentially relevant citations.
- Careful attention should be paid to exclude citations and full-texts that have been retracted post-publication.
- Final inclusion/exclusion decisions should be made after examination of the full-text manuscripts. Reasons for inclusion and exclusion should be recorded. A list of excluded studies should be prepared.
- Language restriction should not be applied in searching or in study selection.
- Duplicate independent assessments of citations and manuscripts should be performed to reduce the risk of errors of judgement in the study selection. In case of disagreements, arbitration by a third reviewer should be used.
- If feasible, an analysis should be undertaken to explore the risk of publication and related biases (see Step 4).

Step 3: *Assessing the quality of the literature*

Step 1
Framing questions
↓
Step 2
Identifying relevant literature
↓
Step 3
Assessing the quality of the literature
↓
Step 4
Summarizing the evidence
↓
Step 5
Interpreting the findings

It cannot be emphasized enough that the quality of the studies included in a systematic review is the 'Achilles' heel' behind its conclusions. Therefore, we should consider study quality at every Step in a review. The quality of a study may be defined as the degree to which it employs measures to minimize bias and error in its *design*, conduct and analysis. We have briefly considered the importance of *study design* as a general marker of study quality when framing questions (Step 1) and selecting studies (Step 2). This approach helps to crudely define the weakest acceptable study *design*, thereby guaranteeing a minimum level of quality.

Once studies of a pre-specified *design* have been selected, an in-depth critical appraisal will allow us to assess the risk of bias and capture the quality of the evidence in a more refined way. Step 3 explains how to develop and use checklists for detailed assessments of selected studies for their quality. These refined and detailed quality assessments will be used in evidence synthesis (Step 4) and interpretation (Step 5). In this way, the quality assessment, also frequently called risk of bias assessment, will help in making judgements about the strength of the evidence collated in a review. In this Step, we will focus on the quality assessment of studies on the effectiveness of *interventions*. The Case studies section of this book gives details of quality assessment of studies on the safety of *interventions* (Case study 2), the accuracy of *tests* (Case study 4), qualitative research (Case study 5), educational effectiveness (Case study 6), adverse effects of drugs (Case study 7) and clinical practice guidelines (Case study 8).

Bias either exaggerates or underestimates the 'true' effect of an *intervention* or *exposure*.

3.1 Study quality or risk of bias assessment checklists

Quality assessment will usually be based on an appraisal of individual aspects of a study's *design*, conduct and analysis – evidence of deficiencies may raise the possibility of bias. Individual quality items put together in the form of a checklist are used in this Step to perform what is often described as a risk of bias assessment. We can find quality items in one of the many *design*-specific published checklists (also called tools or instruments). These have been developed for incorporation in systematic reviews addressing focused questions with collated literature of specific study *designs* (Steps 1 and 2). If such checklists don't exist, published *design*-specific reporting guidelines or guides on critical appraisal of healthcare literature would come in handy. Reporting guidelines focus on transparency of reporting including an emphasis on completely documenting the study methodology in papers. Critical appraisal guides are written for supporting evidence-based practice and provide advice on appraisal of the quality of individual studies according to the nature of

Systematic error (or **bias**) leads to effects departing systematically, either lower or higher, from the 'true' effect.

Random error is due to the play of chance that occurs when a sample of participants is selected to represent a population.

DOI: 10.1201/9781003220039-4

the clinical query, which we delineate when framing our question (Step 1). The items in these published quality checklists, reporting guidelines and critical appraisal guides can be used as a basis for developing a bespoke checklist to perform an in-depth appraisal of the quality of each study included in our review.

There are many published quality assessment checklists for use in systematic reviews; but beware, not all have been developed with scientific rigour. A whole range of quality items is emphasized in the various checklists but some items may not be related to bias. By assigning numerical values to items, some checklists create a scale in an attempt to provide an overall quantitative quality score for each study. Many checklists neatly classify studies into low-or high-quality subgroups based on their compliance with the quality items. If we took a leap of faith and selected one of these published quality checklists for our review, we might find ourselves in trouble. On closer examination, we might find that not all items in the checklist were relevant to our review, and some relevant items were not part of the checklist. For instance, blind *outcome* assessment is emphasized in most checklists. Blinding might be of marginal importance for an unambiguous *outcome* such as mortality, but it is fundamental in the assessment of subjective *outcomes* such as pain. The numerical values assigned to the items for scoring quality may not be suitable for every review; the same is true of the arbitrariness in the criteria recommended for the low–high dichotomy. It is even possible that variation in the choice of checklist might produce different quality assessments for the same studies. Getting worried? Who wouldn't be.

With this background, it should be clear that the *design*-related risk of bias assessment checklists for systematic reviews, reporting guidelines and guides on critical appraisal of studies for evidence-based practice are mostly of a generic nature. Ultimately, it is our responsibility to adapt them to be fit-for-purpose for our review considering our specific questions. If we are lucky, the existing checklist may not need any adaptation, or previous reviews on the same topic may have already developed a suitable study quality assessment checklist. In this situation, re-invention would be pointless. Using an existing checklist or one deployed in previous reviews would also enhance comparability with other literature on our topic. On the other hand, if there are no suitable existing checklists, we will have to develop one. We will need to identify the individual items for assessing quality carefully and judiciously. How can we recognize which items are important for our review? Studies relevant to the review question may be susceptible to specific biases related to the way in which they are conducted and the data they analyse. Therefore, we will have to be prepared to modify or customize a relevant generic quality checklist, including appropriate additional items and deleting irrelevant ones. Our review manuscript would need to give a clear justification for these. Following the approach shown in Box 3.1, the examples in Boxes 3.3 and 3.4 and the demonstrations in the Case studies, we should be able to develop a reasonable study quality assessment checklist for our review.

Box 3.1 Study quality assessment in a systematic review

1. Define the question and the selection criteria:

   - Consider the nature of the questions being posed and the types of relevant *study designs* (Step 1)
   - Determine a basic *study design* threshold which defines the weakest acceptable design for study selection (Step 2)

2. Select a study quality (risk of bias) assessment checklist or develop one
   Identify a suitable existing checklist for your review question. If one does not exist, develop a bespoke quality checklist considering relevant quality items grouped as follows:

   - Generic methodological items related to relevant *study designs* included in the review (usually obtained from published quality checklists, reporting guidelines or critical appraisal guides)
   - Specific issues related to the *participants, interventions* and *outcomes* of the review question may require the creation of new items or customization of the generic items

   Some generic study quality (risk of bias) assessment checklists covered in the Case studies in this book:

Box	Review topic	Quality checklist acronym*
C1.3	Systematic reviews	AMSTAR-2, ROBIS
C2.2	Safety of *interventions*	NOS
C3.3	Effectiveness of *interventions*	ROB-2, ROBINS-I
C4.3	Accuracy of *tests*	QUADAS-2
C8.2	Clinical practice guideline	AGREE II+

   The JBI Manual for Evidence Synthesis provides a range of checklists (jbi.global/critical-appraisal-tools).

   * See the glossary for details.
   + Reporting guidelines may help provide generic quality items.

3. Examine the reliability of checklist use:

   - Assess the reliability of the checklist in a pilot phase before applying it to all the selected studies

4. Incorporate the study quality (risk of bias) assessment throughout the systematic review
   We may use the study quality assessment for all or some of the following:

   - To describe the risk of bias among studies included in a review (Step 3)
   - To explore quality differences as an explanation for the variation in effects from study to study (Step 4)
   - To make decisions regarding pooling the effects observed in included studies (Step 4)
   - To aid in determining the strength of inferences (Step 5)
   - To make recommendations about how future studies could be performed better

3.1.1 Key biases in research addressed by generic quality assessment items

There are many generic biases that reviewers need to consider when developing quality assessment checklists. Bias has been defined as a tendency in research to produce results that depart systematically from the 'true' results. There are several types of biases (also called domains of study quality assessment). Here we shall consider four key biases which impact on the (internal) validity of a study. These are selection bias, performance bias, measurement bias and attrition bias (Box 3.2). Ideally, researchers should try to avoid these biases altogether in primary studies,

Confounding in comparative studies is a situation where the effect of an *intervention* or *exposure* on an *outcome* is distorted due to the association of the *participants* and the *outcome* with another factor, which can prevent or cause the *outcome* independent of the *intervention* or *exposure*.

Box 3.2 Key biases and their relationship to the design and the quality of a study

A study design to assess the effectiveness of interventions

Simple description

A study that allocates (with or without randomization) *participants* to alternative *interventions* and follows them up to determine the effectiveness with which *interventions* improve the *outcome*.

Study flow chart with key biases

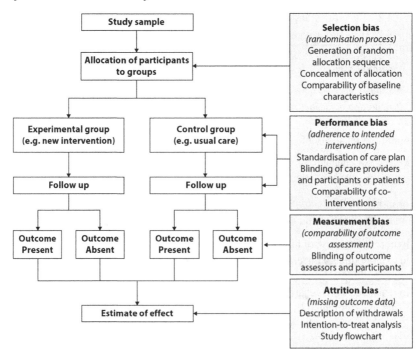

Key biases and their implications for study quality (risk of bias) assessment

Type of bias	Relevant quality items
Selection bias Systematic differences between comparison groups in prognosis or responsiveness to treatment (captured by examining the table of baseline characteristics).	• Generation of random sequence for allocating (a large number of) *participants* to groups • Concealment of allocation from care providers and *participants* (this can be done even in unblinded studies)
Performance bias Systematic differences in care provided apart from the *intervention* being evaluated (captured by examining the table of co-interventions).	• Standardization of care protocol • Blinding of clinicians and *participants*
Measurement bias Systematic differences between comparison groups in how *outcomes* are ascertained.	• Blinding of *participants* and *outcome* assessors
Attrition bias Systematic differences between comparison groups in withdrawals from the study (captured by examining the flow chart of study *participants*).	• Intention-to-treat analysis (or a complete description of withdrawals to allow such an analysis)

See Box 3.4 for generic quality items based on these biases.

ROB-2, the second version of the Cochrane Risk of Bias instrument for assessing the quality of randomized trials included in a systematic review, provides a generic checklist covering the concepts described in this box (methods.cochrane.org/risk-bias-2).

but we know that they don't or can't. Therefore, a very good understanding of these issues must be developed in order to enable us to discover biases during study quality assessment in our review. Our efforts may be made difficult or even impossible due to the poverty of reporting in some studies.

A simple study design for an effectiveness study is shown in Box 3.2. An important requirement for valid results in these studies is that the comparison groups should be similar at the beginning. This is because when there is an imbalance of relevant prognostic features between groups, it becomes difficult for differences in *outcomes* to be confidently attributed to the *intervention* or *exposure*. Technically speaking, this is due to confounding. It is at the time of allocating *participants* to groups that selection bias arises and it is important to check if appropriate measures were designed and implemented to prevent or minimize it. Experimental studies using the random allocation of *participants* (with concealment of allocation sequence) produce comparison groups that are expected to be balanced for known, unknown, and unmeasured prognostic variables. This is the main reason why there has been an emphasis in reviews to focus on randomized trials.

The (internal) **validity** of a study refers to the degree to which its results are likely to be free of **bias**.

Bias either exaggerates or underestimates the 'true' effect of an *intervention* or *exposure*.

Following the allocation of *participants* to groups, performance bias may arise due to unintended *interventions* or co-interventions (e.g. other treatments which are not part of the research). We need to assess if the care plans were standardized and if the researchers and the participants were kept blind to the group allocation during the course of the study. We also need to examine if there was a risk of measurement bias, particularly if the *outcomes* assessed were subjective, and if the participants and researchers involved in ascertaining the *outcomes* were not blind to group allocation. In this way, blinding is important for preventing both performance and measurement bias. Blinding also helps with the control of expectation bias whereby participants, with knowledge of their group allocation, may take co-interventions, drop out, or respond subjectively to outcome measurements.

With respect to multiple *outcomes* among included studies, beware that quality might vary from *outcome* to *outcome*. There may be temptation amongst authors and editors to focus on *outcomes* with statistically significant results, instead of adhering to the order of importance assigned in the original review registration and protocol before starting the study and collecting the data. It is also well known that the planned analyses may be changed with respect to *outcome* measurement, e.g. interchanging scales between binary and continuous, or choice of variables included to adjust for confounding in multivariable models, all just to produce significant p-values. Indeed, statistically non-significant results in pre-specified *outcomes*, *outcome* measurements and analyses may be omitted from published papers. These deviations from planned protocol and data analyses are themselves markers of poor study quality. Prospective registration of studies and publication of their protocols has greatly helped in making these quality assessments, but these are recent initiatives and much of older literature is not evaluable at the same level of rigour.

For preventing attrition bias, an intention-to-treat (ITT) analysis is needed, and it requires data for all *participants*. *Participants*' data are analysed according to their initial group allocation, regardless of whether they fully complied with the *intervention*, changed their *intervention* group during the study or dropped out of the study before its completion. Missing outcome data may have to be imputed in order to permit an ITT. If the selected studies do not perform their analysis in this way, we may be able to do the calculation ourselves, provided a complete description (numbers and reasons) of the withdrawals is available, including information on the people who dropped out, those lost to follow-up and those who have missing outcome data for another reason. If *participants* withdraw from the study and their *outcome* is unknown, there is no satisfactory way to perform ITT analysis. The options available include carrying forward the last *outcome* assessment or imputing the best or worst *outcome* for the missing observations in a sensitivity analysis. Thus, if too many *participants* are lost to follow-up, the analysis may produce biased effects.

Box 3.3 shows how key generic biases can be considered along with biases arising from issues specific to a review concerning the effectiveness

In an **intention-to-treat (ITT) analysis**, participants are analysed grouped according to their initial allocation, regardless of whether they fully complied with the intervention, changed their intervention group after initial allocation, left the study early or have missing outcome data.

Withdrawals are *participants* who do not fully comply with the intervention, cross over and receive an alternative intervention, choose to drop out, are lost to follow-up or have missing outcome data. **Intention-to-treat** analysis with data imputation and an appropriate **sensitivity analysis** is required to deal with withdrawals.

of a treatment for infertility. In this example, good quality research requires that couples have a complete set of investigations for infertility before the *interventions* are provided and that they are followed up for long enough to allow detection of pregnancy. In this way, it would be possible to assess if the treatment led to pregnancies more often than the control without the biasing influences of poor diagnostic workup for infertility and inadequate length of follow-up. These issues are considered along with the generic key biases to produce a checklist for study quality assessment (see Boxes 3.3 and 3.5).

As indicated earlier, the biases related to selection, performance, measurement and attrition are some of the key biases, and the way we present them here pertains mainly to questions about effectiveness. If our question is about the accuracy of tests (Case study 4) or cost-effectiveness (Box 3.4) or some other aspect of healthcare, we will have to consider the biases relevant to these research types for our study quality assessment checklist.

Sensitivity analysis involves the repetition of an analysis under different assumptions to examine the impact of these assumptions on the results. In a primary study where there are **withdrawals**, a sensitivity analysis may involve repeating the analysis, imputing the best or worst outcome for the missing observations or carrying forward the last outcome assessment.

Box 3.3 Example of developing a study quality or risk of bias assessment checklist in an effectiveness review

1) Define the clinical question and the selection criteria

Free-form question: Among infertile couples with subfertility due to a male factor, does anti-oestrogen treatment increase pregnancy rates? (*see the structured question in Box 3.5*)

2) Define the selection criteria

● Nature of question	Assessment of clinical effectiveness
● Study design	Comparative studies (see Box 1.4)
● Study design threshold	Inclusion criterion: Experimental studies
	Exclusion criterion: Observational studies

3) Develop the study quality (risk of bias) assessment checklist

a) Generic methodological quality items for the checklist (*see Box 3.4)

Generation of a random sequence for allocating participants to the interventions

● Adequate
    – computer-generated random numbers or random number tables
● Inadequate
    – use of alternation, case record numbers, birth dates or weekdays
● Unclear or unstated

Concealment of allocation

● Adequate
    – centralized real-time or pharmacy-controlled randomization in unblinded studies, or serially numbered identical containers in blinded studies
    – other approaches with robust methods to prevent foreknowledge of the allocation sequence to clinicians and participants

- Inadequate
  - use of alternation, case record numbers, birth dates or weekdays, open random numbers lists, or serially numbered envelopes (even sealed opaque envelopes can be subject to manipulation)
- Unclear or unstated

Blinding

- Adequate
  - care provider and study participant
- Inadequate
  - care provider or study participant
- Unclear or unstated

Description of withdrawals (to allow an intention-to-treat or ITT analysis)

- Adequate
  - inclusion of all those who dropped out/were lost to follow-up in the analysis
  - numbers *and* reasons provided for missing outcome data in each group
  - description allows analysis following the ITT principle
- Inadequate
  - only numbers (*not* reasons) for missing outcome data provided for each group
  - description does not allow an analysis following the ITT principle
- Unclear or unstated

Coherence with *a priori* trial protocol (not relevant as included trials predated the current prospective trial registration rules)

- Adequate
  - reported all primary and secondary outcomes using the same outcome measurement and the same order as that prospectively registered and written in the published trial protocol or in the protocol version first approved by an ethics committee or in the *a priori* data analysis plan before unblinding outcome data
- Inadequate
  - results reported for outcomes selected possibly due to their statistical significance, instead of adherence to the *a priori* outcomes, outcome measurements or analysis plans
- Unclear or unstated

b) Specific quality items related to the clinical features of the review question

The participants	Complete diagnostic workup for infertility to create groups balanced at baseline
The interventions	No relevant items
The outcome	One year follow-up duration to detect pregnancy as a shorter follow-up duration may not measure the outcome robustly

4) Incorporate the quality assessments into the review

Some examples of the above quality assessment are as follows:

- To describe the quality of studies included in the review (*see Box 3.5*)
- To aid in determining the strength of inferences (*see Box 4.7*)

Box 3.4 Example of developing study quality assessment in a review with multiple questions

1) Define the question and the selection criteria

Free-form question: To what extent is the risk of post-operative infection reduced by antimicrobial prophylaxis in patients undergoing hip replacement and is it worth the costs? (*see the structured question in Box 1.3*)

• Nature of question	Assessment of clinical effectiveness
	Assessment of cost-effectiveness (or efficiency)
	– cost-effectiveness can be assessed by (a) a review of all available full economic evaluations, (b) a review of effectiveness studies in conjunction with any available cost sources, and (c) a secondary economic evaluation using the evidence from the effectiveness review to build an economic decision model. In this example, we consider quality assessment for option (a).
• Study design	Effectiveness: Experimental studies
	Cost-effectiveness: Full economic evaluations
• Study design threshold	Effectiveness (see Box 1.4)
	– inclusion criterion: Experimental studies
	– exclusion criterion: Observational studies
	Cost-effectiveness (*see glossary*)
	– inclusion criterion: Full cost-effectiveness analyses
	– exclusion criterion: Partial economic evaluations

2) Develop the study quality assessment checklist

Some generic quality items for checklists

- Clinical effectiveness review
  - random allocation of participants to groups
  - concealment of allocation sequence
  - pre-specified criteria for eligibility of participants
  - similarity of groups at baseline regarding prognostic factors
  - blinding of care providers, participants and outcome assessors
  - an intention-to-treat analysis
- Cost-effectiveness review
  - a comprehensive description of alternative interventions
  - identification of all important and relevant costs and outcomes for the interventions
  - use of established evidence of clinical effectiveness, i.e. intervention known to improve outcome
  - costs and outcomes measured accurately and valued credibly
  - costs and outcomes adjusted for differential timing
  - an incremental analysis of costs and outcomes
  - sensitivity analyses for uncertainty in costs and outcomes

Box 3.5 Example of tabulation and graphic presentation of study quality (risk of bias) assessment

Free-form question: Among infertile couples with subfertility due to a male factor, does anti-oestrogen treatment increase pregnancy rates?

Structured question

• The participants	Couples with subfertility due to a male factor (low sperm count)
• The interventions	Anti-oestrogen treatment (clomiphene citrate or tamoxifen) for the male partner
	Comparator: Placebo, no treatment, or vitamin C
• The outcomes	Pregnancy (critical)
• The study design	Experimental studies

Tabulation of study quality (risk of bias) assessment

Information about quality items coded according to explicit and transparent definitions can be placed in columns with the studies in rows (sorted according to the year of publication).

Author	Year	Randomization Sequence generation	Concealment	Blinding	Description of withdrawals	Participants' complete workup	Outcome measurement with 1-year long follow-up	Rank order of quality*
Roonberg	1980	Unstated	Unstated	Unclear	Adequate	Adequate	Inadequate	3
Abel	1982	Unclear	Unclear	Inadequate	Adequate	Unclear	Inadequate	4
Wang	1983	Unclear	Unclear	Inadequate	Unclear	Adequate	Adequate	6
Torok	1985	Unclear	Unclear	Unclear	Unclear	Inadequate	Adequate	5
Micic	1985	Unclear	Unclear	Inadequate	Unclear	Inadequate	Inadequate	9
AinMelk	1987	Unclear	Unclear	Unclear	Unclear	Inadequate	Inadequate	8
Sokol	1988	Adequate	Adequate	Adequate	Unclear	Adequate	Adequate	1
WHO	1992	Adequate	Adequate	Adequate	Adequate	Adequate	Inadequate	2
Karuse	1992	Unclear	Unclear	Inadequate	Unclear	Inadequate	Inadequate	7

* See text in Section 3.4 and Box 3.3 *for an explanation.*

Bar chart of study quality (risk of bias) assessment

Information on quality is presented as 100% stacked bars. Data in the stacks represent the number of studies meeting the quality criteria.

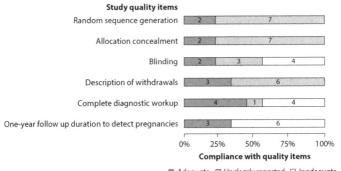

Based on Arch Intern Med 1996; **156**: 661–6, doi: 10.1001/archinte.1996.00440060089011.

See Box 4.1 for advice on the construction of tables.

See Box 4.7 for use of study quality assessment in exploring heterogeneity.

3.1.2 Integrity concerns

Research integrity, by its general definition, emphasizes the concept of 'trust' instilled in scientific findings through responsible research conduct based on ethics and professionalism. It covers all aspects of a study from its conception to publication, including design, conduct and analysis. Thus, quality assessment essentially captures its integrity as evaluable by systematic assessment of the risk of bias in the included studies. Typically, this is done through evaluation of what is reported in the published papers without access to the original protocols and the raw data.

Think for a moment about why we need to perform study quality assessment? Well, by undertaking these assessments, implicitly we declare that we can't really place much weight on 'trust' in the system of science production and publication. The system is imperfect, though speaking about it explicitly would take the courage of the innocent to shout out 'the emperor has no clothes'. Once it is accepted that the authors, peer-reviewers, editors and others concerned all have difficult-to-manage conflicts of interests, it is easy to see why post-publication concerns may be raised about studies. These would need to be investigated and in case of findings of questionable research conduct or outright misconduct, an expression of concern may be issued by journals or the paper may be retracted. As no good system for removing retracted papers from circulation exists, they remain searchable (Step 2) and may continue to be cited and (mis)used.

It goes without saying that systematic reviews, for their own integrity, would be best to avoid including studies with questionable, fabricated or falsified data. Reviewers should be mindful that such literature does not get included in their review, but what can they practically do about it. This topic, at the time of writing, is not backed by properly developed tools for post-publication integrity evaluations. The least reviewers can do is to look out for prospective registrations, public documentation of study protocols and statistical analysis plans, and data, if shared. They should also look out for concerns raised in literature searches (Step 2) about included studies through examination of their citations in letters to the editors published as correspondence and commentaries in the journals. Independent online platforms such as PubPeer (pubpeer.com) also offer a forum for post-publication peer-review and communication of concerns. In case of any issues about the integrity of included studies, new reviewers should consult their seniors for advice.

Research integrity requires compliance with ethical and professional principles, standards and practices by individuals or institutions. **Fabrication** is making up data and using them as if genuine. **Falsification** is manipulation of data in a way that they are inaccurately represented.

3.2 Study quality assessments in reviews with a mixture of *designs*

In the past, there has been a strong emphasis for reviews to focus on a single *study design* of the highest quality, i.e. randomized controlled trials (Box 1.4). However, reviewers soon realized that for many important questions, studies of high-quality *designs* were often not available

(Case study 2) or they were scarce (Case study 3). This is either because no one undertook such studies in the past or if they did try, it was not practicable or ethical to conduct them. When there is a dearth of studies with a high-quality *design*, it is not uncommon for reviews to include a mixture of *designs* to summarize the available evidence. This approach carries implications for evidence synthesis (Step 4) and interpretation (Step 5). However, reviews including studies with multiple *designs* need not be confusing, particularly if due attention can be given to the quality assessment issues.

When using the approach described in Box 3.1, we might find that in some reviews, where the question demands studies of various designs to be included, the quality assessment will not be so straightforward. A mixture of studies with different designs may become part of a review because more than one design is needed to address the same question or because more than one question is to be addressed. Case study 3 presents an example where studies of both experimental (randomized and non-randomized) and observational (cohort study with concurrent controls) designs are included in a review to address a question about effectiveness. Here it is possible to develop and use a single checklist for quality assessment (Boxes C3.3 and C3.4). Some reviewers prefer to use separate checklists for different designs and this is the most reasonable approach in some situations; for example, when a review addresses two separate but related questions, e.g. about clinical effectiveness and efficiency of an *intervention*. This is like having two reviews in one. Here different quality assessments will have to be developed for the different study *designs* relevant to the two questions, as shown in Box 3.4.

3.3 Reliability of the study quality checklist in a review

The evaluation of quality items is very often affected by vague and ambiguous reporting in the selected studies. In order to avoid subjectivity and errors when extracting information about quality, the review protocol should provide a clear description of how to assess quality. This would mean designing data extraction forms with clear and consistent coding of responses. Ideally, the forms should be piloted using several reviewers and a sample of studies to assess the reliability of the study quality assessment process. Pilot testing might identify confusion about the extraction and coding instructions, which would then need to be clarified – a more explicit system of coding would improve the inter-reviewer agreement. When disagreements arise, the resolution procedure deploying consensus and arbitration should be pre-specified.

In the past, people have suggested blinding the reviewers to the names of the authors, institutions, journals and year of publication when assessing quality. This should avoid bias as judgements about quality may be unduly influenced by these factors. Therefore, some reviewers go to great lengths to have such identifying information masked before examining

Effectiveness is the extent to which an *intervention* (therapy, prevention, diagnosis, screening, education, social care, etc.) produces beneficial *outcomes* under ordinary day-to-day circumstances. Effectiveness trials tend to be pragmatic with adequate sample sizes for clinically relevant *outcomes*, intention-to-treat analyses and an emphasis on generalizability when defining *participant* selection criteria.

Efficacy is the extent to which an *intervention* can produce beneficial *outcomes* under ideal circumstances.

Efficiency (cost-effectiveness) is the extent to which the balance between inputs (costs) and outputs (*outcomes*) of *interventions* represents value for money.

the manuscripts. However, the cumbersome and time-consuming procedures required to produce blinded papers have not been shown to
impact on the conclusions of reviews and unmasked independent quality
assessment by more than one reviewer should be sufficient. By now it
should be quite clear that it is unwise to undertake a review without
co-authors.

3.4 Using study quality assessments in a review

Having developed our study quality assessment checklist and extracted
the relevant data on the risk of bias, we are ready to integrate this information into our review (Box 3.1). How would we describe the quality of
the studies? There are many imaginative ways of presenting information
about how the studies included in a review have complied with the quality
items. Examples of quality descriptions are shown in the case studies. We
may start by describing how many studies meet the various quality criteria and support this with graphs, e.g. using stacked bar charts (Box 3.5).
However, tabulation of the information on quality items for each one of
the included studies is the clearest way to describe quality (Box 3.5).

One difficult issue in quality assessment is that of ranking studies
according to their quality. A simple way is to rank studies according to
the proportion of total items they comply with. When studies satisfy the
same proportion of quality items, but are deficient in different areas,
there is a problem. Here the deficient areas should guide us about the
rank: studies with deficiencies in areas with a greater potential for bias
(e.g. lack of concealment of allocation) should be ranked lower than those
with deficiencies in areas with a smaller risk (e.g. deficiencies in allocation sequence generation). The weighting of items has been proposed
but there are no agreed weighting schemes that apply universally. This is
because the importance of quality items varies from topic to topic. For
example, blinding is highly crucial in studies with subjective *outcomes*,
but not so much in those with objective *outcomes*.

Reviewers have to use their judgement when ranking studies according to quality in the context of their topic. For example, in a review
concerning the effectiveness of a treatment for infertility (Box 3.5),
two studies (Sokol and WHO) comply with five out of six quality items.
Sokol is 'unclear' about its description of withdrawals and WHO has not
followed *participants* up for 1 year for capturing *outcomes* (in fact they
only followed up for 8 months). If we feel that adequacy of follow-up is
more important than lack of clarity about the description of withdrawals,
then we can rank Sokol higher than WHO. This subjectivity cannot be
removed from reviewing, so it is important that judgements are made
before the results of the studies are known and are reported transparently. This example should also make it clear that there are limits to how
detailed judgements can be. Often it is impossible to have a sensible
ranking of studies according to quality and one may have to settle for a

more crude categorization, e.g. high-*versus*-low quality studies, as in Case study 2. Having performed study quality assessments in a sensible (and unbiased) manner, one can confidently proceed to data synthesis (Step 4), interpretation of results and generation of inferences (Step 5) where the variation in the quality of the selected studies may have important implications. We see examples of how the strength of evidence in a review is linked to study quality assessment in Box 5.3 and Case study 7.

Writing tips for systematic review authors

- **Abstract:** Specify the study *design(s)* selected, provide the study quality assessment checklist, give a brief description of the overall risk of bias among the included studies and ensure that the conclusion reached is bound within any limitations placed by the study quality assessment.
- **Methods:** In the data extraction or study quality assessment subsection, describe with reference the study quality assessment checklist chosen for risk of bias assessment. Give an overview of the domains, quality items and their coding, making clear how these relate to your review question and specifying any adaptations or customizations made with justification. Give details of how an overall judgement about individual study quality was reached. Also describe how quality assessments were initially piloted and subsequently undertaken in duplicate, and what was done to resolve disagreements amongst reviewers through discussion or arbitration. If agreement statistics are computed, these are typically described under statistical analysis. The data synthesis subsection describes how study quality assessment was incorporated into the statistical analysis. Be mindful that if the review includes quality assessments separately for a different *outcome*, the text of a manuscript should specify the *outcome* when describing methods and results.
- **Results:** Dedicate text concerning study quality assessment when describing study characteristics. Any agreement statistics computed concerning study quality assessment are reported here too. Tabulate the study quality assessments per study (in rows) including individual items and overall assessment (in columns). If there are too many studies to fit the table comfortably in the main text, summarize its findings in a diagram, usually Figure 2 based on a 100% stacked bar chart giving both study numbers and percentages for each quality item and overall assessment (easily constructed using the graph function in a spreadsheet like Excel). The long table underpinning the figure can be included as an appendix to go with the manuscript. Present the results of the data synthesis taking into account study design and quality assessment.
- **Figure:** Give the quality assessment figure a detailed title for it to stand alone. Simply stating 'Figure 2: Study quality assessment' is

IMRaD is an acronym that refers to the section headings used in writing the main manuscript text, i.e. I-Introduction, M-Methods, R-Results, a-and, D-Discussion, of a systematic review paper for submission to a peer-reviewed journal. See Case study 10 for tips, tricks and unwritten rules for convincing journal editors and peer-reviewers to publish your article.

insufficient. Clarify which review the quality assessment pertains to including elements of the review question, e.g. 'Figure 2: Quality of included studies in the systematic review of anti-oestrogens for male infertility'. Include detailed legends to explain the figure, e.g. numbers in the stacked bars represent the number of studies meeting the quality criteria and the axis represents the percentage compliance. In footnotes give the location of the source data, e.g. the table or appendix number, and name the quality assessment checklist with its bibliographic reference.

- **Discussion:** Give a brief description of the overall risk of bias among the included studies as part of the initial paragraph concerning the main findings. Describe the review's strengths and limitations taking into account the study quality. Ensure that the review's conclusion is bound within any limitations placed by the quality assessment (a review that synthesizes garbage cannot be expected to deliver gold as its output!).

Summary of Step 3: Assessing the quality of the literature

Key points about appraising review articles

- Examine the abstract and the methods section to see if a study quality (risk of bias) assessment has been undertaken.
- Has a *design*-based threshold been used as a criterion for study selection? (Step 2)
- Has a more detailed assessment of the selected studies been carried out? Are the quality items appropriate for the question? Check the results section with the tables and figures to see how much variation in quality there is between studies.
- Is the variation in quality an explanation for heterogeneity? Is meta-analysis appropriate given the quality? Have subgroup analyses or meta-regression been carried out to evaluate the impact of variation in study quality? (Step 4)
- Has the evaluation of the strength of the collated evidence been linked to study quality (risk of bias), not just to p-values? (Step 5)

Key points for conducting reviews

- Obsession with quality is the 'Achilles' heel' of all research studies and reviews. Study quality (risk of bias) assessment plays a role in every Step of a proper systematic review.
- Question formulation (Step 1) and study selection criteria (Step 2) should have study *design* components in them to determine the minimum acceptable level of study quality.
- For a more refined quality assessment of selected studies, checklists should be developed which consider the generic issues relevant to the study *design* aspects of the review question. These items may be derived from existing *design*-based quality checklists, reporting guidelines and critical appraisal guides.

- It is important to customize the generic checklists considering issues relevant to the *participants, interventions* and *outcomes* specific to the review question. Considering these specific issues, the existing generic items may be modified or deleted and new relevant items may be added to the quality checklists.
- Prospective registrations, public documentation of study protocols and statistical analysis plans, and data sharing are increasingly being implemented for ensuring research integrity. Seek all available information to help in the detailed study quality (risk of bias) assessment.
- Prepare to first pilot and then fully undertake the risk of bias assessment for each included study in duplicate to capture each quality item with explicit coding in a spreadsheet. This will help produce detailed tables and figures that present the study quality data transparently.
- These detailed quality (risk of bias) assessments will be used for describing the selected studies, exploring an explanation for heterogeneity (Step 4), making informed decisions regarding the suitability of meta-analysis (Step 4), assessing the strength of the collated evidence (Step 5) and making recommendations for future research.

Step 4: *Summarizing the evidence*

Step 1
Framing questions
↓
Step 2
Identifying relevant
literature
↓
Step 3
Assessing the quality
of the literature
↓
Step 4
Summarizing the
evidence
↓
Step 5
Interpreting the
findings

Collating the findings of studies included in a review requires more than just tabulation and meta-analysis of their reported results. It requires a deeper exploration and an in-depth analysis, for which the findings need to be presented in a clear way. We need to evaluate whether the observed effects of *interventions* are consistent among the included studies and if not, why not? We need to assess if a statistical combination of individual effects (meta-analysis) is feasible and appropriate. These analyses allow us to generate meaningful conclusions from the reviews. This Step covers the basics of producing evidence summaries in systematic reviews, limiting the discourse to questions about the reported effects of *interventions* or *exposures* on binary *outcomes*. Once the principles are understood, they can be applied with appropriate tailoring to other question types (Case studies 4, 5 and 6).

4.1 Description of data contained in the included studies

To begin with, a descriptive summary of the findings of studies included in a review is required. In simple terms, the objective of this initial exercise is to present (in a meaningful way) the information about the studies' characteristics (*participants, interventions* and *outcomes*), their *design* and quality, and their effects. There is no need to use any advanced statistics at this stage. We may use tables, figures and simple computations, such as proportions, relative risks, etc., which allow us to glance at the evidence and glean the differences between studies, either in their characteristics (*participants, interventions* and *outcomes*) or in their *designs* and quality as well as in their effects. This is a crucial part of evidence synthesis; it will help us gain a deeper understanding of the evidence and should prevent errors in interpretation. It will also enhance the transparency of our data synthesis.

When faced with large amounts of data to be summarized, tabulation can be a daunting task. The process of carrying out the tabulations should follow from the review question. The nature and complexity of the tables depend a great deal on how many studies are included and how much data needs to be displayed from each. The decisions about the structure of the tables should be guided by what we considered to be important issues at the time of question formulation and what, in our judgement, could produce a variation in effects as outlined in Step 1. So, for example, information may be tabulated with studies in rows grouped according to a characteristic of the *participants*. Then information on *interventions, outcomes* and effects for each study could be summarized succinctly (Box 4.1). Information on *outcomes* should make clear the importance attached to each *outcome* separately.

Effect is a measure of the association between an *intervention* or *exposure* and an *outcome*. The term **individual effects** means effects observed in individual studies included in a review. **Summary effect** means the effect generated by pooling individual effects in a meta-analysis.

Box 4.1 Tabulating information from studies included in a systematic review

Suggested steps

1. Place features related to participants, interventions and outcomes in columns.
2. Consider what subgroups of participants and interventions there are among the included studies.
3. Consider the outcomes, their measurement and their importance.
4. Consider if studies need to be subclassified according to study designs and quality.
5. Populate the cells in the table with information from studies along rows in subgroups.
6. Sort studies according to a feature that helps to understand their results (e.g. a characteristic of a participant or intervention, the rank order of quality, the year of publication, etc.).
7. Give table titles that permit it to stand alone. Simply stating 'Table 1: Study characteristics' is insufficient. Include elements of the review question to identify the table as part of the specific review, e.g. 'Table 1: Characteristics of studies included in the systematic review of antimicrobials for chronic wounds'. Use footnotes liberally to explain the contents of the table such that the need to refer to the main text is obviated.

An example of tabulation of studies in a review of antimicrobials for chronic wounds

This is only a brief tabulation. Detailed tables can be found in the published review available at doi: 10.1046/j.1365-2168.2001.01631.x

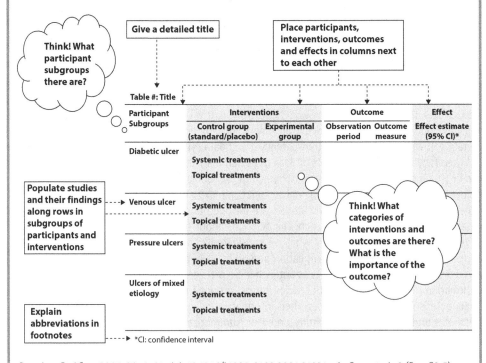

Based on Br J Surg 2001; **88**: 4–21, doi: 10.1046/j.1365-2168.2001.01631.x *in Case study 3 (Box C3.5).*

Sometimes tables will end up with too many columns to fit on one page. In this situation, it is often helpful to break down the tabulation into several tables. We may produce one detailed table of *participant* characteristics and relevant prognostic factors; another table may include details of *interventions* and yet another for details of *outcomes*. The features of *study designs* and study quality assessment may be presented in a separate table or a figure (Box 3.5). Preparation of tables is often laborious and time-consuming, but without them we cannot understand the results of the included studies. Once the hard work is done, a quick scan through these tables should allow us, and more importantly others, to judge how studies differ in terms of *participants*, *interventions*, *outcomes*, *design* and quality.

At this stage, we should also compute and tabulate the effects reported in each one of the studies along with their confidence intervals (Box 4.2). This will help us examine the direction and magnitude of effect among the individual studies. By direction of effect, we mean either benefit or harm. By magnitude, we mean how much benefit or how much harm. Box 4.3 shows how to evaluate the direction and magnitude of effect graphically in a Forest plot.

Box 4.2 Estimation of effects observed in individual studies included in a systematic review

Measures of effect

An effect is a statistic which provides a measure of the strength of the relationship between an intervention and an outcome, e.g. relative risk (RR), odds ratio (OR) or risk difference (RD) for binary data; mean difference or standardized mean difference for continuous data; and hazard ratio for survival data (see glossary). Statistical significance tells us nothing about the magnitude of the effect. Effect measures help us to make judgements about the magnitude and clinical importance of the effects. The term individual effects means the effects observed in individual studies included in a review. Summary effect means the effect generated by pooling individual effects in a meta-analysis.

Computing effect measures for binary outcomes in individual studies

Computing point estimates of effects is relatively simple, as shown below. It is a comparison of the frequency, i.e. the risk or the odds, of the outcomes in the comparison groups. This comparison could be a ratio (RR and OR) or a difference (RD, or its inverse, the number needed to treat or NNT). These are relative and absolute measures of effect, respectively. It is worth noting that ratio measures cannot be calculated if there are no events or outcomes present in the control group. They cannot be calculated also if all participants in the experimental group have experienced the event. With several studies to compute effects for, and to estimate confidence intervals for, every effect makes manual calculation tedious. We would suggest you use a statistical software package. We have generally used RevMan, the Cochrane Collaboration's review management software, to compute and present results in this book (cochrane.org).

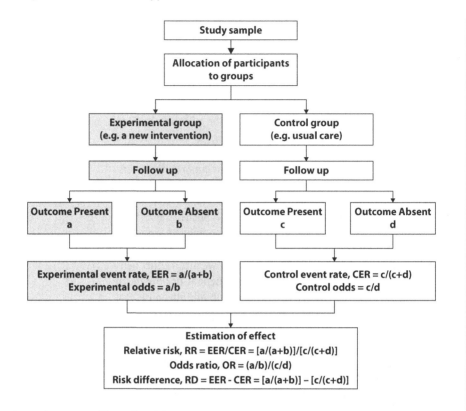

Choosing an effect for binary outcomes

The choice depends on the ease of interpretation and statistical properties of the effect measure. Clinicians prefer relative risk (RR) and the number needed to treat (NNT) – which is the inverse of risk difference (RD) – because they are intuitive. OR may be more considered suitable for statistical modelling. OR and RD are not sensitive to the reversibility of the outcome classification. RR and OR are relative measures of effect, compared to RD which is an absolute measure of effect. The summary RR value generated from meta-analyses can be challenging as their meaningful clinical application depends on the knowledge of baseline rates in the *setting* where the results are to be applied (see Step 5). We will often be faced with OR in the medical literature. From these, we can generate NNTs for interpretation as shown in Box 5.4.

Box 4.3 Summarizing the effects observed in studies included in a systematic review

Forest plot

This is a commonly used, easy to understand, graphical display of individual effects observed in studies included in a systematic review (along with the summary effect if meta-analysis is used, as in Box 4.4). For each study, a box representing the point estimate of the effect lies in the middle of a horizontal line which represents the confidence interval of the effect.

When using relative risk (RR) or odds ratio (OR) as the effect measure, the effects are usually plotted on a log scale. This produces symmetrical confidence intervals around the point estimates. A vertical line drawn at an RR or OR value of 1.0 represents 'no effect'. For desirable outcomes (e.g. pregnancy among infertile couples), RR or OR value > 1.0 indicates that the experimental intervention is effective in improving that outcome compared to the control intervention. However, most reviews report undesirable outcomes (e.g. death), and then RR or OR values < 1.0 indicate an advantage for the experimental group. When using mean difference, the value 0 indicates 'no effect'. A confidence interval overlapping the vertical line of 'no effect' represents the lack of a statistically significant effect.

Description of effects and their uncertainty in a systematic review

Free-form question: Among infertile couples with subfertility due to a male factor, does anti-oestrogen treatment increase pregnancy rates? *(see the structured question in Box 3.5)*

The effects observed among nine studies

The effects are summarized as RR and OR, sorted by the year of publication. Effect values > 1.0 indicate an advantage for the treatment group compared to the control, i.e. pregnancy rates improve with anti-oestrogen treatment.

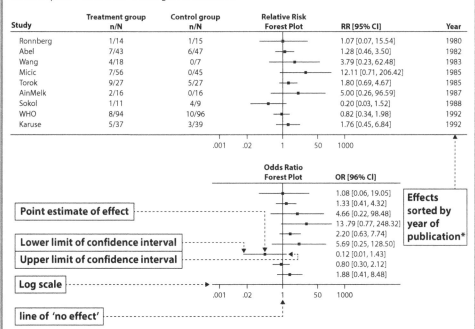

Study	Treatment group n/N	Control group n/N	Relative Risk Forest Plot	RR [95% CI]	Year
Ronnberg	1/14	1/15		1.07 [0.07, 15.54]	1980
Abel	7/43	6/47		1.28 [0.46, 3.50]	1982
Wang	4/18	0/7		3.79 [0.23, 62.48]	1983
Micic	7/56	0/45		12.11 [0.71, 206.42]	1985
Torok	9/27	5/27		1.80 [0.69, 4.67]	1985
AinMelk	2/16	0/16		5.00 [0.26, 96.59]	1987
Sokol	1/11	4/9		0.20 [0.03, 1.52]	1988
WHO	8/94	10/96		0.82 [0.34, 1.98]	1992
Karuse	5/37	3/39		1.76 [0.45, 6.84]	1992

.001   .02   1   50   1000

Odds Ratio Forest Plot — OR [96% CI]

1.08 [0.06, 19.05]
1.33 [0.41, 4.32]
4.66 [0.22, 98.48]
13.79 [0.77, 248.32]
2.20 [0.63, 7.74]
5.69 [0.25, 128.50]
0.12 [0.01, 1.43]
0.80 [0.30, 2.12]
1.88 [0.41, 8.48]

.001   .02   1   50   1000

Labels in figure:
- **Effects sorted by year of publication***
- **Point estimate of effect**
- **Lower limit of confidence interval**
- **Upper limit of confidence interval**
- **Log scale**
- **line of 'no effect'**

*Based on Arch Intern Med 1996; **156**: 661–6, doi: 10.1001/archinte.1996.00440060089011.*

Review manager software is used to compute effects and produce graphics. It is developed by the Cochrane Collaboration and is available as a free download following registration. Technical support is provided only for Cochrane reviewers. Web-based versions of software may become standard in the future.

* See Box 4.7 for a Forest plot with individual studies sorted according to the rank order of quality and subgrouped by low and high quality.

A simple tabulation of numerical results, like the one shown in Case study 3 (Box C3.5), is not easy to assimilate at a glance. Therefore, it is worth examining the effects graphically (Box 4.3). These graphic summaries would help us make qualitative judgements about the effects of *interventions*, particularly about the direction, magnitude, precision and variability of individual effects. Occasionally, this may produce a surprise: a conclusion about effectiveness may be reached solely from a qualitative examination of the observed effects without the need for statistical analysis, particularly if there are numerous high-quality studies with consistent and large effects. In this situation, a quantitative synthesis (meta-analysis) may not add anything to our inferences. However, often the effects will not be precise enough because of a small sample size in individual studies. The graphic display will give us a good idea about effectiveness, but this will not be sufficient to generate inferences. Here, meta-analysis will be useful, as it will improve the precision of the effect by statistically combining the results from individual studies – but first we need to assess if the effects vary from study to study (heterogeneity) and if it is sensible to undertake a meta-analysis.

One aim of a data description is to assess the extent of the evidence in order to plan statistical analyses. We should have planned our analyses for heterogeneity and meta-analysis in advance, and included them in the prospective registration and review protocol (Step 1). Armed with information from the tables, we should be able to assess the feasibility of the planned analyses. We will be able to see if data on clinically important *outcomes* are available for the *interventions* we wanted to compare. We may become aware of additional issues of importance, which were not known at the planning stage. If we decide to pursue these issues, we should be honest about reporting them as *post hoc* analyses and we should be conscious of the problems of spurious significance associated with them. Our enquiry might be limited due to lack of data or due to missing information on important issues. It might be useful to contact the authors of individual studies before proceeding further; alternatively, we could plan a sensitivity analysis to take account of the uncertainties due to missing or unclear information.

4.2 Investigating differences in effects between studies

There are usually some differences between studies in the key characteristics of their *participants*, *interventions* and *outcomes* (clinical heterogeneity), and their *study designs* and quality (methodological heterogeneity). These are discovered during the tabulation of information from the studies. These variations in study characteristics and quality are likely to have some influence on the observed effects. Investigation of heterogeneity is about this variation of effects between studies and its reasons.

Point estimate of effect is its observed value in a study.

Confidence interval is the imprecision in the point estimate, i.e. the range around it within which the 'true' value of the effect can be expected to lie with a given degree of certainty (e.g. 95%). The width of the confidence interval is related to the sample size and the numbers with the outcome within the comparison groups.

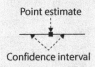

Point estimate

Confidence interval

The **direction of effect** indicates a beneficial or a harmful effect. The point estimate of effect tells us about the direction and magnitude of the effect.

The **precision of effect** relates to the degree of uncertainty in the estimation of the effect. The confidence interval tells us about precision. The wider the confidence interval, the lower the precision of the estimate of the effect.

Sensitivity analysis involves the repetition of an analysis under different assumptions to examine the impact of these assumptions on the results.

We may begin exploring for the possibility of heterogeneity of effects between studies by studying the tables we produced earlier. However, we will probably get a better idea about heterogeneity by visually examining the Forest plot for variations in effects (Box 4.3). In general, if the point estimates of effects lie on one side of the 'line of no effect', then the *interventions* can be expected to produce the same qualitative effect, either benefit or harm. If the point estimates are located on both sides of the 'line of no effect', then they could produce beneficial and harmful effects (as in Box 4.3). Clearly, this should raise suspicion about heterogeneity. We should also see if the confidence intervals of the effects overlap with the summary effect. If they do, as in Box 4.4, then it is more likely that any differences in the point estimates of effects are merely due to chance or indicate only limited heterogeneity, which is unavoidable.

Formal statistical tests for heterogeneity examine if the observed variability in effects is above that which is expected to occur by chance alone. The chi-square test for heterogeneity among the effects shown in Box 4.4 has a *p*-value of 0.36 – well above the conventional threshold of $p < 0.05$. These tests tend to have low power, so they might miss important between-study differences in effects. It has therefore been suggested that a less stringent threshold of $p < 0.1$ should be used to statistically assess heterogeneity. The formal assessment with the *p*-value has a serious drawback. The underlying chi-square statistic which leads to the *p*-value, let's call it Q, has no intuitive meaning. Q increases as the number of included studies, k, increases. To have a more appropriate tool for the assessment of heterogeneity, $I^2 = (Q - (k - 1))/Q$ has been introduced. I^2 is interpreted as the proportion of the existing variability due to heterogeneity between studies. I^2 ranges between 0% and 100%; 0% indicates no observed heterogeneity, and larger values show increasing heterogeneity. Values of 25%, 50% and 75% may be taken to represent low, moderate and high levels of heterogeneity. With I^2 dependence on the number of included studies is avoided. However, I^2 still hinges on the precision of the studies, or, in other words, on the size of the studies. This limits the use of I^2 when comparing values across meta-analyses with different study sizes.

Assessment of heterogeneity is a challenge in the synthesis of studies. There remain many disputes between methodologists about the interpretation of heterogeneity statistics and details of these are beyond the scope of this book. A reasonable approach would be to evaluate both informal, non-statistical assessment of heterogeneity (e.g. with the Forest plot) and the I^2 statistic without reliance on *p*-values alone. Whenever we suspect substantial heterogeneity, we should seek an explanation, whether or not heterogeneity is statistically confirmed. We will turn to exploring reasons for heterogeneity shortly, but first we take a look at the basics of meta-analysis.

Question components
The participants: A clinically suitable sample of patients

The interventions: Comparison of groups with and without the intervention

The outcomes: Changes in health status due to interventions

The study design: Ways of conducting research to assess the effect of interventions

Heterogeneity is the variation of effects between studies. It may arise because of differences in key characteristics of their *participants*, *interventions* and *outcomes* (clinical heterogeneity), or their study *designs* and quality (methodological heterogeneity). It also may arise because of the play of pure chance (statistical heterogeneity).

Power is the ability of a test to statistically demonstrate a difference when one exists. When a test has low power, a larger sample size is required; otherwise, there is a risk that a possible difference might be missed.

I^2 is a statistic ranging from 0% to 100% that gives the percentage of total variation across studies due to heterogeneity.

Box 4.4 Summarizing the effects using meta-analysis

Forest plot of individual and summary effects

Effects observed in individual studies are plotted along with the summary effect. For each study, the point estimate of effect is a box of variable size according to the weight of the study in the meta-analysis. The summary effect is plotted below the individual effects using a different graphic pattern, e.g. a filled diamond (the width of the diamond represents the confidence interval and the centre of the diamond represents the point estimate).

An example meta-analysis using fixed and random effects models

The example shown below is based on the question and the effects (relative risk, RR) described in Box 4.3. Compared to the fixed effect models, the random effects models produce a wider confidence interval around the summary effect because they take into account between-study variability. They also preferentially weight smaller studies, which have more varied effects than larger studies.

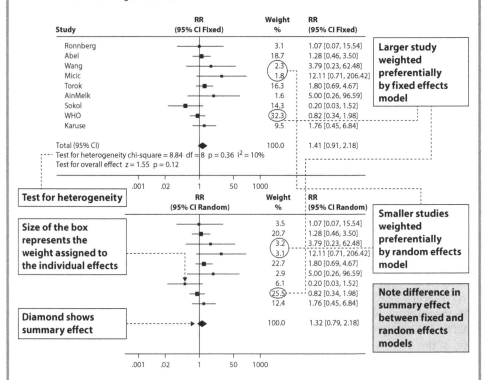

Based on *Arch Intern Med* 1996; **156**: 661–6, doi: 10.1001/archinte.1996.00440060089011.

Review manager software is used to compute effects and produce graphics.

See Box 4.7 for subgroup meta-analysis.

4.3 Meta-analysis (quantitative synthesis) of effects observed in studies

As indicated earlier, individual studies may be far too small to produce precise effects and so meta-analysis can improve precision by combining them statistically. First, we must determine if meta-analysis is at all possible, and if so, whether it would be appropriate. By examining the tables produced for describing the studies, we will be able to determine if the data necessary to perform a meta-analysis are available. Sometimes meta-analysis will just not be feasible; for example, when there are important differences between the studies in terms of *participants*, *interventions*, *outcomes*, *design* and quality, it would be senseless to try to estimate a summary effect (as in Case study 3). A systematic review does not always have to have a meta-analysis! In addition, by examining for differences in effects between studies, we will be able to determine whether or not the studies are too heterogeneous to be sensibly combined. We should proceed with meta-analysis only if the studies are similar in clinical characteristics and methodological quality, and are homogeneous in effects.

In a meta-analysis, in simple terms, the effects reported in the included studies are pooled to produce a weighted average effect of all the studies – the summary effect. Individual effects across studies are collated to ensure that the *intervention* group within each study is compared to the control group in the same study. Thus, in a meta-analysis of experimental studies, the benefit accrued by randomization (with allocation concealment) is preserved when the individual results are pooled. For pooling, each study is weighted according to some measure of its importance, e.g. a method that gives more weight to more informative studies (often larger studies with precise effect estimates) and less weight to less informative studies (often smaller studies with imprecise effect estimates) is used. In most meta-analyses, this is achieved by assigning a weight to each study in inverse proportion to the variance, expressing precision, of its effect. An example meta-analysis is shown in Box 4.4.

It is important to be familiar with the finer points concerning pooling individual effects in a meta-analysis because we will be faced with them regularly when reading or conducting reviews. During a meta-analysis, it is essential to check how robust our summary effect is to the variation in statistical methods. There are two concepts to keep in mind: the 'fixed effect' and 'random effects' statistical models.

A fixed effect model estimates the average effect assuming that there is a single 'true' underlying effect. It assumes that all studies are estimating the same 'true' effect. A random effects model assumes that there is no single underlying value of the effect, but there is a distribution of effects depending on the studies' characteristics. The differences between effects are considered to arise from between-study variation

Meta-analysis is a statistical technique for combining the individual effects of a number of studies addressing the same question to produce a summary effect. This book focuses on meta-analyses conducted using reported study-level data. **Individual participant data meta-analysis** using the raw data collected in the included studies is an advanced technique not covered in this book. **Network meta-analysis**, another advanced technique that may be used in systematic reviews addressing broad questions comparing multiple interventions, is also not covered in this book.

and the play of chance (random variability). A random effects model weights smaller studies proportionally higher than a fixed effect model when estimating a summary effect. This phenomenon may exaggerate the impact of smaller studies and could be detected using publication bias analysis (Section 4.8).

Random effects models incorporate the variance of effects observed between the studies to compute the weight of individual studies. Hence, when there is heterogeneity, a random effects model produces wider confidence intervals of the summary effect compared with a fixed effect model. Therefore, it can be argued that the fixed effect model may give undue precision to the summary effect (spuriously narrow confidence interval) if there is significant unexplained heterogeneity between the studies. It is worth noting that in absence of significant statistical heterogeneity, results of the random effects model tend to produce a summary effect with confidence interval close to the one produced by the fixed effects model. This makes it more prudent to assume the random effect model is the desirable model for data synthesis. In the example meta-analysis shown in Box 4.4, summary effects generated with both fixed and random effects models are demonstrated. In practice, both statistical models may be used to assess the robustness of the statistical synthesis, but if we have to make a choice, we should do this *a priori* and not after we have been biased by knowledge of the results.

4.4 Clinical heterogeneity

Differences in the characteristics of the studies with respect to *participants, interventions* and *outcomes* can provide useful answers regarding heterogeneity and can help in interpreting the clinical relevance of the findings. The exploration of these differences can be facilitated by constructing the summary tables in such a way that potential explanations for differences in effects can be more easily identified. During question formulation (Step 1), we would have identified important issues that could produce a variation in effects (see examples in Box 1.3). Based on this information, we may stratify the studies into subgroups according to *participants, interventions* and *outcomes* sets. The differences in effects in the various subgroups of studies can then be explored.

If there are many studies in our review, the differences in effects may also be examined statistically, as shown in Box 4.5. We can perform a meta-analysis of subgroups of studies and additionally examine if the effects are consistent within the subgroups. Advanced statisticians could also determine the statistical significance (p-value) of the difference in the effect between subgroups (see meta-regression below). We should be aware that investigations into the reasons for heterogeneity must be interpreted with caution. As with statistical tests for detection of heterogeneity, tests for evaluating its reasons also have limited power, so they may miss a relationship. Another problem is that if subgroup analyses are carried out, some might be spuriously significant, a problem inherent in

Variance is a statistical measure of variation measured in terms of deviations of the individual observations from the mean value. It quantifies the precision or the error of an estimation made using a sample of participants.

The **inverse of variance** of observed individual effects is often used to weight studies in statistical analyses used in systematic reviews, e.g. meta-analysis, meta-regression and funnel plot analysis. This weighting makes the individual studies with lower variance (i.e. with less error in the estimation of individual effects) have more importance in the calculation of the average pooled effect.

multiple analyses of any type. Therefore, examination of the explanation for heterogeneity should be planned for a small number of study characteristics for which there is a strong suggestion of a relationship with the size of the effect. In addition, the choice of subgroups should be made in advance (Step 1). It is good to be cautious – from examining the tables we generated earlier, we might become aware of issues and possible relationships we had not anticipated. The temptation would be to undertake further subgroup analyses that were not originally planned. These *post hoc* analyses should be avoided. If we cannot resist the temptation, they should be clearly identified and their findings should be interpreted cautiously. They should not be used to guide clinical practice, but they can be used to generate hypotheses for testing in future research.

Where substantial heterogeneity is present and clinical reasons for it can be found, an overall meta-analysis may be unnecessary. In this situation, meta-analysis should be restricted to clinically relevant subgroups where a variation in effect was originally anticipated. This approach will aid in the clinical interpretation and application of the review's findings as highlighted by the example shown in Box 4.5.

Box 4.5 Exploring clinical heterogeneity

Subgroup analysis

Free-form question: Do home visits improve the health of elderly people?

Structured question

● The participants	Elderly people in various age groups
● The interventions	Home visits of various intensities and frequencies
● The comparator	Usual care
● The outcomes	Mortality, functional status and nursing home admissions
● The study design	Experimental studies

Delineation of various subgroups (*considering the detailed question structure in Box 1.3*)

Subgroups	1 Age-based subgroups	2 Assessment intensity-based subgroups	3 Follow-up frequency-based subgroups
● The participants	Elderly people in various age groups	Elderly people	Elderly people
● The interventions	Home visits	Home visits of various assessment intensities	Home visits of various frequencies of follow-up
● The comparator	Usual care	Usual care	Usual care
● The outcomes	Mortality (critical)	Functional status (critical)	Nursing home admissions (important)

Subgroup meta-analyses

A vertical line in the centre of the diamond indicates the point estimate of the summary relative risk (RR) for each subgroup of studies with particular characteristics. The width of the diamond represents the confidence interval of the summary RR for each subgroup. RR values of < 1.0 represent an advantage for the intervention group compared to the control.

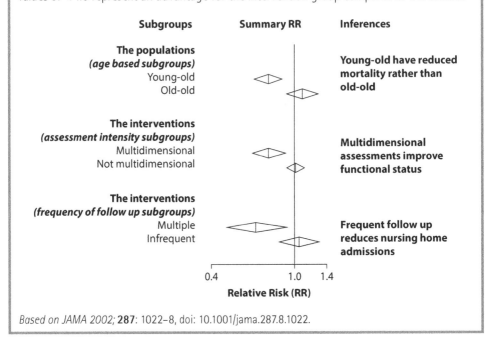

Based on *JAMA 2002;* **287**: 1022–8, doi: 10.1001/jama.287.8.1022.

4.5 Methodological heterogeneity

We should also find out if *design* and quality differences among studies appear to be associated with variation in their effects. This is important not only to explore reasons for heterogeneity, but also to assess the strength of the evidence (Step 5).

   Hopefully, the *study design* will have been used as one of the selection criteria (Step 2). This way studies of poor *design* would have been removed and the review would have focused on studies of a minimum acceptable quality from the outset. So why should there be a fuss about the quality of a review's component studies? In many reviews, depending on the type and amount of available literature, it is inevitable that selection criteria specifying the *study design* will allow the inclusion of studies of methodologically inferior *designs* (Step 2). Even when search and selection focus on robust *study designs*, there will be some variation in quality between studies. This happens because the devil about quality is in the detail: the 'gross' hierarchies of *study designs* used for study selection do not capture finer points about quality which are important for the validity of the results.

Hopefully, we would have performed detailed study quality assessments and discovered the variation in quality between studies (Step 3). During study synthesis, we should gauge if quality has an association with the estimation of effects as part of the exploration for heterogeneity and its sources. The reason for being concerned about study quality is that if we find different individual effects among studies of different quality, we can no longer trust the overall summary effect. If high-quality studies produce conservative estimates of effect, our inferences would also have to be conservative.

We may have got some idea about the relationship between quality and effects by tabulating the relevant information on quality and effects together. In fact, where studies of different *designs* are included in a review, we should tabulate the studies subgrouped according to *design*. In this situation, if a meta-analysis is (mistakenly) undertaken using studies of different *designs*, there is a risk that biased summary effects may be produced due to undue weighting of studies that are inferior in *design*. In an attempt to counter such a bias, the idea of weighting studies in proportion to their quality (rather than size or precision as described earlier) has been suggested. However, no agreed standards exist for producing such weights, so we should abandon this idea. Sometimes the only feasible approach will be a descriptive evidence summary, particularly if there are no subgroups of studies of a similar quality, but if there are, use a subgroup meta-analysis.

A meta-analysis should only be contemplated within subgroups of studies of the same *design* and inferences should be based on the effects observed among studies of superior *design*. As shown in Box 4.6, we might find that studies of superior *designs* do not show an association

> The **quality** of a study depends on the degree to which its design, conduct and analysis minimize **biases**.

> **Bias** either exaggerates or underestimates the 'true' effect of an *intervention* or *exposure*.

Box 4.6 Using study design to gauge the strength of inferences

Free-form question: Is exposure to benzodiazepines during pregnancy associated with malformations in the newborn baby? (*also see Box 1.2*)

Structured question

● The participants	Pregnant women
● The exposures	Benzodiazepines in early pregnancy
● The comparator	No exposure
● The outcomes	Major malformations in the newborn baby
● The study design	Observational studies with cohort and case-control designs (*see Box 1.4*)

Summary of evidence

There was statistically significant heterogeneity in the overall analysis. Overall summary odds ratio (OR) suggested a trend towards an association between exposure to benzodiazepines and the risk of major malformations in the newborn baby. We use OR in this analysis because among studies with a case-control *design*, it is not possible to compute risk and relative risk.

Exploring the impact of study design on the effects observed in the review

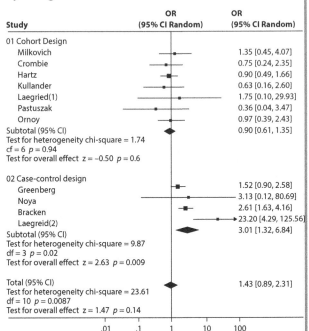

Subgroup analysis stratified according to study design

The association between exposure to benzodiazepines in pregnancy and major malformations is only supported by the subgroup of case-control studies (where there is heterogeneity). These studies are of a more inferior design than cohort studies. Among the sub-group of studies with cohort design (where there is no heterogeneity) there is no association.

Note: OR values >1.0 indicate an association of malformations with exposure to benzodiazepines compared to no exposure.

Study	OR (95% CI Random)
01 Cohort Design	
Milkovich	1.35 [0.45, 4.07]
Crombie	0.75 [0.24, 2.35]
Hartz	0.90 [0.49, 1.66]
Kullander	0.63 [0.16, 2.60]
Laegried(1)	1.75 [0.10, 29.93]
Pastuszak	0.36 [0.04, 3.47]
Ornoy	0.97 [0.39, 2.43]
Subtotal (95% CI)	0.90 [0.61, 1.35]

Test for heterogeneity chi-square = 1.74
cf = 6 p = 0.94
Test for overall effect z = –0.50 p = 0.6

Study	OR (95% CI Random)
02 Case-control design	
Greenberg	1.52 [0.90, 2.58]
Noya	3.13 [0.12, 80.69]
Bracken	2.61 [1.63, 4.16]
Laegreid(2)	23.20 [4.29, 125.56]
Subtotal (95% CI)	3.01 [1.32, 6.84]

Test for heterogeneity chi-square = 9.87
df = 3 p = 0.02
Test for overall effect z = 2.63 p = 0.009

Study	OR (95% CI Random)
Total (95% CI)	1.43 [0.89, 2.31]

Test for heterogeneity chi-square = 23.61
df = 10 p = 0.0087
Test for overall effect z = 1.47 p = 0.14

Naïve inference without considering study design
Exposure to benzodiazepines in pregnancy is possibly associated with major malformations in the newborn baby.

Inference considering study design
Exposure to benzodiazepines in pregnancy is *not* associated with major malformations in the newborn baby.

Based on Dolovich et al. BMJ 1998; **317**: *839–43.*

RevMan software is used to compute effects and produce graphics.

See Box 4.4 for summarizing effects using meta-analysis.

between *exposure* and *outcome* when studies of inferior *designs* do. Even when a review focuses on studies of a single *design*, there may be variation in effects according to quality. Often the relationship between quality and effect would result in heterogeneity, but this is by no means the rule. If the studies' effects were stacked in decreasing order of quality in a Forest plot, the relationship would become apparent. For example, an increase in the point estimate of effect may be observed as the quality deteriorates, as shown in Box 4.7.

We should explore the relationship between study quality and effects even when heterogeneity is not statistically demonstrable, because effects among high-quality studies may be different from those among low-quality studies (Box 5.3). There is some controversy about how to do this. Some experts consider it preferable to perform a subgroup analysis, stratifying the studies according to their compliance with individual quality items, but this has the disadvantage of increasing the number of subgroups (see Case study 4), which in turn carries the risk of spurious statistical significance. Alternatively, quality scores (composed of the quality items) may be used to stratify studies, but the scoring systems are usually not well developed (Step 3). If there

---

Box 4.7 Using study quality to gauge the strength of inferences

Free-form question: Among infertile couples with subfertility due to a male factor, does anti-oestrogen treatment increase pregnancy rates? (*see the structured question in Box 3.5*)

Summary of evidence (based on the review summaries in Boxes 4.3 and 4.4)

There was no statistically significant heterogeneity in the overall analysis. Summary relative risk (RR) suggested a trend towards an increase in pregnancy rate among couples treated with anti-oestrogens.

Exploring the impact of study quality on the effects observed in the review

Forest plot with effects stacked in decreasing order of quality*

For high-quality studies there is a trend towards harm from treatment. As the quality of studies decreases this trend reverses and the possibility of benefit emerges.

Subgroup analysis stratified according to quality*

The beneficial trend in the overall meta-analysis is supported only by low-quality studies. High-quality studies suggest a trend towards harm, i.e. decrease in pregnancy rates, with treatment.

Note: Relative risk (RR) values >1.0 indicate an advantage for anti-estrogen treatment compared to control.

See Box 3.5 for detailed quality assessment of individual studies and rank order.

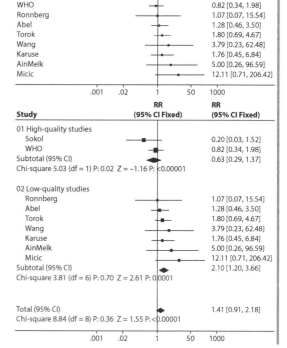

Study	Relative Risk	RR [95% CI]
Sokol		0.20 [0.03, 1.52]
WHO		0.82 [0.34, 1.98]
Ronnberg		1.07 [0.07, 15.54]
Abel		1.28 [0.46, 3.50]
Torok		1.80 [0.69, 4.67]
Wang		3.79 [0.23, 62.48]
Karuse		1.76 [0.45, 6.84]
AinMelk		5.00 [0.26, 96.59]
Micic		12.11 [0.71, 206.42]

.001   .02   1   50   1000

Study	RR (95% CI Fixed)	RR (95% CI Fixed)
01 High-quality studies		
Sokol		0.20 [0.03, 1.52]
WHO		0.82 [0.34, 1.98]
Subtotal (95% CI)		0.63 [0.29, 1.37]
Chi-square 5.03 (df = 1) P: 0.02 Z = –1.16 P: <0.00001		
02 Low-quality studies		
Ronnberg		1.07 [0.07, 15.54]
Abel		1.28 [0.46, 3.50]
Torok		1.80 [0.69, 4.67]
Wang		3.79 [0.23, 62.48]
Karuse		1.76 [0.45, 6.84]
AinMelk		5.00 [0.26, 96.59]
Micic		12.11 [0.71, 206.42]
Subtotal (95% CI)		2.10 [1.20, 3.66]
Chi-square 3.81 (df = 6) P: 0.70 Z = 2.61 P: 0.0001		
Total (95% CI)		1.41 [0.91, 2.18]
Chi-square 8.84 (df = 8) P: 0.36 Z = 1.55 P: <0.00001		

.001   .02   1   50   1000

> **Naïve inference without considering the quality**
> Anti-oestrogen therapy seems to have a trend towards a beneficial effect among infertile couples with subfertility due to a male factor.
>
> **Inference considering study quality**
> Anti-oestrogen therapy has *no* beneficial effect among infertile couples with subfertility due to a male factor.

Based on Arch Intern Med 1996; **156**: 661–6, doi: 10.1001/archinte.1996.00440060089011.

RevMan software is used to compute effects and produce graphics.

See Box 3.5 for a detailed description of quality.

See Box 4.3 for a Forest plot with studies sorted according to the year of publication.

See Box 4.4 for summarizing effects using meta-analysis.

is a good correlation between studies with regard to compliance (and non-compliance) with a number of quality items, it may be sensible to stratify studies into high- and low-quality subgroups based on compliance with most of the quality items (Box 4.7). This approach would reduce the number of subgroup analyses and minimize the risk of spurious findings.

4.6 Meta-regression

As a complementary procedure to subgroup analysis for exploring heterogeneity we have a technique called meta-analytic regression (or meta-regression in short). Both procedures – subgroup analysis and meta-regression, are intimately related. We should touch on it briefly, mainly with a view to helping us with critical appraisal. From a bird's-eye view, we can say that meta-regression is the statistical test to demonstrate whether there is a significant difference between the effects estimated in two subgroups (e.g. studies with a high risk of bias compared to the subgroup of studies with low risk of bias). More generally, we can test associations of categorical variables (that make the subgroups) as well as with continuous variables (e.g. age of participants, dose of the drug, etc.). Put simply, this technique fits a linear regression model for examining the influence of study characteristics and quality on the size of individual effects observed among studies included in a review. In this way, it searches for the unique contribution of different variables towards an explanation for heterogeneity. These characteristics are known as covariates or effect modifiers. As a difference from standard regression analysis, in this case, each study has a different weight depending on the precision of its effect estimation. This weight is mainly driven by the study sample size and the frequency of events.

Confounding in meta-regression is a situation where the effect of an intervention is associated simultaneously with multiple characteristics of studies included in a meta-analysis. It occurs when studies being pooled are different with respect to characteristics that are themselves correlated. For example, studies with a particular participant characteristic such as age may be correlated with methodological quality. In this situation, the observation of higher effects in studies of older people may be linked to poor study quality. Adjustment for confounding when exploring reasons for heterogeneity requires multivariable meta-regression analysis.

Meta-regression does have a downside – it suffers from the risk of what is described in regression analysis as 'overfitting'. This arises because reviews often only have a small number of studies and a large number of varia-bles are available for inclusion in the model. In this situation, if a regres-sion model is used, it will lead to spurious findings. So, beware! As a rule of thumb, we may test the association of one covariate for every 10 studies included in the review. This limits seriously the number of study characteris-tics that can be explored for their relationship with heterogeneity. Left with not many options, it is common to fit univariate meta-regression models rather than multivariate models. This reduces the risk of 'overfitting', but it leaves to subjective judgment the evaluation of confounding that arises because the characteristics of the studies could be correlated. Think, for example, a scenario in which studies at higher risk of bias tended to recruit older patients. If an association appears between age and the effect of the intervention, we could not disentangle whether this association is due to the participants' mean age or because of the poor quality of the studies (Box 4.8). In large systematic reviews, multivariable meta-regression can productively explore both clinical and methodological reasons for heterogeneity, adjusting for confounding. The most powerful way to

---

Box 4.8 Meta-regression plots for exploring reasons for heterogeneity

Meta-regression plots

Participants' age
- Continuous variable (age in years).
- Effects in older participants appear to be better.
- Effect may be related to participants' age, but this may be because of the influence of higher risk of bias among studies in older people.

Methodological quality of studies
- Categorical variable (low vs high risk of bias).
- Studies at high risk of bias have higher effect sizes.
- Study quality will likely contribute to heterogeneity.

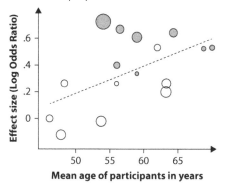

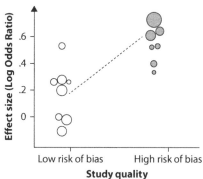

Weight of studies is represented by the size of the circle. Larger circles have greater precision. Filled circles have a higher risk of bias in study quality assessment.

Based on a hypothetical example.

assess between-study differences is based on an analysis using individual participant data from the included studies. However, this remains an aspiration rather than a goal for most reviews.

4.7 Meta-analysis when heterogeneity remains unexplained

Hopefully, the studies included in our review will not have any obvious heterogeneity. If we do encounter it, hopefully our exploration for the reasons behind the heterogeneity will bear some fruit. However, in many reviews, there will be no explanations, neither clinical nor methodological. In this situation, one might say that heterogeneity remains unexplained despite a sensible exploration. This may be because the number of studies in a review is not large enough to allow a powerful analysis to decipher the reasons behind differences in effects between studies. Now, do we or do we not perform a meta-analysis? There is no simple answer.

We should ask ourselves what is to be gained by meta-analysis. Can we not interpret the studies' findings with tabulation and Forest plots of individual effects? The temptation would be to attribute the heterogeneity to chance variation between studies and then undertake a meta-analysis using a random effects model. This approach wrongly assumes that a random effects model accounts for the variation between studies that cannot be explained by other factors. This is particularly tricky when the number of studies is small, thus producing a poor estimation of the dispersion (i.e. variance) of the underlying distribution of effects. If we do succumb to this temptation (which happens far too often), proceed with caution. Make sure to look for and exclude funnel asymmetry (Box 4.9), a factor indicative of publication and related biases. Otherwise, a random effects model may produce biased summary effect estimates. In addition, our interpretation of the summary effect should be cautious as heterogeneity limits the strength of the evidence collated in reviews (Step 5). We must examine to see if the overall summary effect and the effects of the high-quality subgroup of studies are, by and large, consistent. Even when there is no apparent reason for heterogeneity, the results of high-quality studies may be different. In this way, quality becomes a factor in the assessment of the strength of evidence (Step 5).

Publication bias is said to arise when the likelihood of publication of studies and thus their accessibility to reviewers is related to the significance of their results regardless of their quality.

4.8 Exploring for publication and related biases

How can we be sure that our review does not suffer from publication and related biases? Hopefully, a systematic approach has been used to track down studies, whether they are published or not (Step 2). Hopefully, the

Box 4.9 Funnel plots to explore for publication and related biases

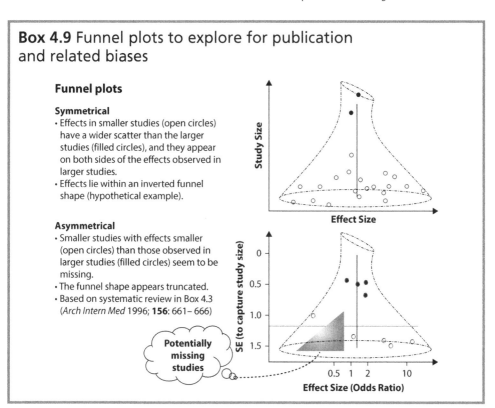

Funnel plots

Symmetrical
- Effects in smaller studies (open circles) have a wider scatter than the larger studies (filled circles), and they appear on both sides of the effects observed in larger studies.
- Effects lie within an inverted funnel shape (hypothetical example).

Asymmetrical
- Smaller studies with effects smaller (open circles) than those observed in larger studies (filled circles) seem to be missing.
- The funnel shape appears truncated.
- Based on systematic review in Box 4.3 (*Arch Intern Med* 1996; **156**: 661– 666)

Potentially missing studies

search has particularly focused on capturing those studies that are less accessible, e.g. through searching multiple databases, and has not used language restrictions in study identification. Hopefully, the cast net is wide enough to capture all relevant studies (or at least an unbiased sample of the relevant literature). However thorough the literature search is, there cannot be any guarantees. But there can be some comfort (or discomfort) from formal *post hoc* assessment for publication and related biases in a review.

A simple, in many cases too simple, but commonly used method of exploring for these biases is based on the so-called 'funnel plot' analysis. To perform this analysis meaningfully, numerous studies, including some large studies, are required. The accepted rule of thumb is not to proceed with this analysis unless at least 10 studies are included. As shown in Box 4.9, it is a scatter plot of individual effects that are observed among studies included in a review against some measure of study precision (e.g. study size, the inverse of the variance). If all the relevant studies ever carried out are included in our review, the scatter of data points in the plot can be expected to lie within a symmetric funnel shape. The funnel is inverted when the y-axis is taken to represent study size (or inverse of the variance), as in Box 4.9. This is because there is a wider range of effects among smaller studies compared to the effects observed among larger studies, owing to less precision in

Variance is a statistical measure of variation, measured in terms of the deviation of the individual observations from the mean value.

The **inverse of variance** of observed individual effects is often used to weight studies in the statistical analyses used in systematic reviews, e.g. meta-analysis, meta-regression and funnel plot analysis.

smaller studies. In this situation the funnel, therefore, is symmetrical and we can have more confidence that publication and related biases are unlikely in our review. If the funnel is truncated (sometimes called banana-shaped), a group of studies may be missing from our review. Usually, missing studies are small in size with different effects from those observed in the large studies included in our review. Such omissions are unlikely to be due to chance alone and they make the funnel asymmetrical. Publication bias is just one of a host of related reasons for funnel asymmetry, including location bias, English language bias, database bias, citation bias, multiple publication bias, the poor methodological quality of small studies and clinical heterogeneity (e.g. small studies in high-risk participants), to name a few. The multiplicity of reasons, and the difficulty in separating them from each other, has led to the use of the term small-study-effect rather than publication bias. Whatever the reason, our confidence in the findings of the review will be limited if there is a truncation of the funnel.

A number of statistical tests are available to examine if funnel asymmetry is likely to be due to chance. These are outside the remit of this book, but some advice will be helpful for critical appraisal of reviews. The shapes of funnel plots vary according to the measures of effect and study size, and statistical tests for asymmetry often don't give consistent results. So, to avoid overinterpretation, funnel plot analyses should only be considered exploratory in nature. If it is any consolation, the true extent of publication and related biases may never be known.

Writing tips for systematic review authors

- **Title:** If meta-analysis is a key part of the review, then include this term in the title.
- **Abstract:** State the meta-analytic methods used. Report the effect estimates giving 95% confidence intervals and I^2 statistics.
- **Methods:** In the data synthesis subsection, provide the meta-analytic methods and software programs used. Outline the planned subgroup analyses and meta-regression models for exploration of reasons for heterogeneity. Report transparently any modifications to the planned analyses. Explore for risk of publication and related biases.
- **Results:** Report included study data along with the individual and overall effect estimates giving 95% confidence intervals and I^2 statistics. Give findings of exploration of reasons for heterogeneity and of funnel asymmetry analyses. There may be too many tables and figures to accommodate them all in the main text; judiciously select a few and move the rest to appendices.
- **Tables and figures:** Give detailed titles that permit them to stand alone. Abbreviations should be accompanied with full descriptions even if they have been described in the abstract and the main text. Use footnotes liberally to explain anything that could assist in understanding their contents without the need to refer to the main text.

IMRaD is an acronym that refers to the section headings used in writing the main manuscript text, i.e. I-Introduction, M-Methods, R-Results, a-and, D-Discussion, of a systematic review paper for submission to a peer-reviewed journal. See Case study 10 for tips, tricks and unwritten rules for convincing journal editors and peer-reviewers to publish your article.

- **Discussion:** Give a brief description of the main findings without using numerical results as part of the initial paragraph of the discussion. Describe the review's strengths and limitations taking into account the risk of publication bias, clinical and methodological heterogeneity, and statistical precision of the findings. Ensure that the review's conclusion is bound within any limitations placed by these.
- **Supplementary material:** Data sharing, in addition to what should be transparently presented in tables, figures and appendices, is increasingly a requirement for systematic review publications. Provision of the painstakingly extracted data on the risk of bias and 2×2 tables from the individual included studies into electronic spreadsheets may soon become obligatory. Prepare data files along with statistical analysis codes and outputs for uploading as the supplementary material.

Summary of Step 4: Summarizing the evidence

Key points about appraising review articles

- Examine the abstract, methods and results sections to see if heterogeneity of effects is evaluated.
- Was the exploration for heterogeneity planned in advance?
- Is variation in clinical characteristics of the studies an explanation for heterogeneity?
- Is variation in study design and quality an explanation for heterogeneity?
- Are the numerical data of included studies reported?
- Are measures of heterogeneity like I^2 provided and results interpreted in the light of the observed heterogeneity?
- Is meta-analysis appropriate in the light of information gathered on heterogeneity and its reasons?
- Is there a risk of publication and related biases?

Key points about conducting reviews

- The aim of this Step is to collate and summarize the findings of studies included in a review.
- Data synthesis consists of tabulation of study characteristics and quality as well as their numerical data and individual effects. This permits the use of statistical methods for exploring differences between studies and combining their effects (meta-analysis) appropriately.
- Tabulation of evidence helps in assessing the feasibility of planned statistical syntheses and improves overall transparency.
- Exploration of heterogeneity and its sources should be planned in advance.
- Exploration of clinical heterogeneity should be based on a small number of study characteristics for which there is a strong theoretical basis for a relationship with an estimation of an effect.

- Exploration of methodological heterogeneity should consider factors for which there is a strong theoretical or empirical basis for suspecting a relationship with bias.
- The following questions should be considered prior to embarking on meta-analysis: Is meta-analysis feasible given clinical heterogeneity? Is meta-analysis feasible given the variation in study quality? Is meta-analysis feasible given the statistical heterogeneity?
- If an overall quantitative summary is not feasible, a subgroup meta-analysis might be feasible and could provide clinically useful answers.
- Meta-regression provides a useful tool for exploring clinical and methodological reasons for heterogeneity in a single analysis.
- If feasible, funnel plot analysis should be undertaken to explore for the risk of publication and related biases.

Step 5: *Interpreting the findings*

Step 1
Framing questions
↓
Step 2
Identifying relevant literature
↓
Step 3
Assessing the quality of the literature
↓
Step 4
Summarizing the evidence
↓
Step 5
Interpreting the findings

Deciphering the salience of a review's findings is a scientific, not artistic, pursuit. The ultimate purpose of a review is to inform decision-making and allow knowledge to underpin the action. The big question at the end of a systematic review is 'how can one go about making decisions with the collated evidence?' However, the task of generating meaningful and practical answers from reviews is not always easy. We will cover some of the key issues that aid sensible and judicious interpretation of the evidence, avoiding both over- and under-interpretation.

By the time our review is nearing completion or after having read someone else's review, we may think that we already know the meaning of the findings. But what are the main findings? Is the evidence strong? It isn't the *p*-value that determines the real significance of the findings. How much trust can we have in the results of the review? How can we generate inferences and recommendations for current clinical practice as well as for future research? The answers to these questions may not be as straightforward as one might think in the first instance.

A related issue is that there is no standardization of reporting of strengths and weaknesses of the collated evidence in published systematic review articles. This makes it difficult for readers to assess the trustworthiness of the bottom line given in published papers. This Step advises on how the key findings, the strength of their underpinning evidence and their implications for practice all come together in drawing the review's conclusion. This is usually done in writing the discussion section of the manuscript's main text (Box C10.3). Some journals may ask you to give the limitations of the evidence within the abstract. This approach allows for transparency, caveats spelt out upfront, when summing up the review.

This Step describes explicit and replicable ways to determine the strength of the evidence collated in a review for generating clinically meaningful and trustworthy bottom lines that aid in the application of research into practice. The approach outlined is used for generating formal recommendations in guidelines. It will also assist us as review authors to opine on what clear recommendations emerge directly from our evidence synthesis in the discussion section of the manuscript, and what areas of uncertainties there are that define the evidence gaps.

The Grading of Recommendations Assessment, Development and Evaluation (**GRADE**) working group is an informal collaboration that aims to develop a comprehensive methodology for assessing the strength of the evidence collated in systematic reviews and for generating recommendations from evidence in guidelines (gradeworkinggroup.org).

5.1 Strength of the evidence

How do we gauge the strength of the evidence? First, it is important to recognize that language concerning the concept of overall evidence strength varies in the literature, e.g. GRADE working group vocabulary for this is evidence certainty. Trustworthiness, in the general sense, is what we wish to capture formally in Step 5. This attribute depends on the evaluation of the strengths and weaknesses of the review in each one of its Steps, e.g. how well did it comply with the key points on appraising reviews at the end of each Step in this book:

- Is there evidence available on critical and important *outcomes* for the *participants* and *intervention* of interest described in the question?
- Are the searches adequate?
- Is there a risk of publication and related biases?
- Is the *design* and methodological quality of the included studies good enough (i.e. is the risk of bias low enough)?
- Are the results consistent from study to study?
- Are there enough data for precise estimation of the effect (i.e. are the confidence intervals narrow enough)?
- Are the observed effects of substantial clinical, not just statistical, significance?

We have formulated a structured question focused on clinically relevant *outcomes*. We have to compare how well the evidence matches the components of the question. Were the study *participants* sicker, older or from a different setting? Are *interventions* replicable in our workplace? We have thought about *outcomes* relevant to patients and have focused our review on core critical and important *outcomes* (Step 1). Are results available for these critical and important *outcomes*? The principal findings should relate to these. Other findings should be considered secondary.

Having undertaken a thorough literature search (Step 2), we have examined the results for publication bias and other related biases (Box 4.9). We have considered the design and quality of studies included in the review (Step 3; Box 3.5). We have explored the observed effects of the individual studies for (in)consistency (Step 4). We have probed whether certain *participant* features such as the severity of the disease or the setting (Box 4.5), *intervention* features such as treatment intensity or timing (Box 4.5) or methodological features such as study design or study quality (Boxes 4.6 and 4.7) are associated with a larger or reduced size of the relative effect. We have inspected the confidence intervals around the effect estimates to evaluate (im)precision.

The effect is a measure of the association between *exposures* or *interventions* and *outcomes*.

The direction of effect indicates a beneficial or a harmful effect. The point estimate of effect tells us about the direction and magnitude of the effect.

The precision of effect relates to the degree of uncertainty in the estimation of effect that is due to the play of chance. The confidence interval tells us about precision. The wider the confidence interval, the lower the precision of the estimate of the effect.

Question components
The participants: A suitable sample of participants

The exposures: Comparison of groups with and without the exposure

The outcomes: Changes in health status due to interventions

The study design: Ways of conducting research to assess the effect of interventions

Publication bias is said to arise when the likelihood of a study being published, and thus its accessibility to reviewers, is related to the significance of its results regardless of their quality.

Clinically relevant *outcomes* directly measure what is critical and important to patients in terms of how they feel, what their function is and whether they survive. Such outcomes are crucial for decision-making.

Core *outcomes* are a group of critical and important outcomes on which there is consensus that they should be measured and reported. Systematic reviews are used to create a long list of outcomes which is then reduced to a core outcomes set through surveys collating evaluations of patients and practitioners.

Box 5.1 Levels of the strength of evidence collated in a review

The strength of evidence describes the extent to which we can be confident that the estimate of an observed effect, i.e. the measure of association between *exposures* or *interventions* and *outcomes* assessed in the review, is correct for critical and important *outcomes*.

High strength of evidence:	We are very confident that the true effect lies close to the observed effect.
Moderate strength of evidence:	We are moderately confident that the true effect is likely to be close to the observed effect, but there is a possibility that it could be substantially different.
Low strength of evidence:	Our confidence in the observed effect is limited. The true effect may be substantially different from that observed.
Very low strength of evidence:	We have very little confidence in the observed effect. The true effect is likely to be substantially different from that observed.

Having explored in-depth the above issues individually, we ultimately need to look at them collectively to make a judgement about the overall strength of the evidence. This judgement should be arrived at in an explicit manner. It would be wise to stop for a moment and consider what we mean by the term **strength of evidence**: In the context of systematic reviews, the strength of the evidence describes the extent to which we can be confident that the estimate of an observed effect is correct for critical and important *outcomes*. The judgements on the strength of the evidence can be formally classified as being of high, moderate, low or very low level (Box 5.1).

5.1.1 Assigning a level of strength to evidence

We begin the process of assigning a level of strength to evidence by evaluating the study design (Box 1.4). As a default rule, evidence from experimental design is initially assigned a high level of strength while that from observational design is assigned a low level. Appraisal of key issues concerning directness of evidence in relation to the question, publication bias, methodological quality (risk of bias) of included studies and heterogeneity and precision (confidence intervals) of results is then employed to lower the initially assigned level of strength by one or two levels. This depends, as shown in the examples below, on how much the critical appraisal of key issues alters the confidence in the observed effect.

The **point estimate** of effect is its observed value in a study.

The **confidence interval** is the imprecision in the point estimate, i.e. the range around it within which the 'true' value of the effect can be expected to lie with a given degree of certainty (e.g. 95%). The width of the confidence interval is related to the sample size and the numbers with the outcome within the comparison groups.

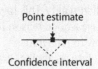

Point estimate

Confidence interval

Strength of evidence describes the extent to which we can be confident that the estimate of an observed effect is correct for critical and important *outcomes*. It takes into account the directness of outcome measure, study design, study quality (risk of bias), heterogeneity, imprecision (confidence interval width) and publication bias (this is not an exhaustive list).

One has to explicitly consider how good the methodological quality of included studies has to be for evidence to be valid? How consistent should the effects be across studies to be homogeneous? How large should an improvement in effect be for it to be relevant for clinical practice? When is a confidence interval narrow enough to be called precise? Addressing these questions involves judgement, which requires a mixture of methodological and clinical expertise. Whatever the judgement, it should be explicit and transparent so that others can make sense of the reasoning employed to assign levels of strength of evidence.

Consider Case study 3 for instance, where the included studies are of experimental design. To begin with, one may consider the strength of evidence to be at a high level. If the review on antimicrobial therapy in chronic wounds only reported the *outcome* reduction in histologically documented inflammation, most would agree there would be difficulties in translating results based on this surrogate into practice. This is because we would prefer to base practice on results from data on a clinically relevant *outcome* like complete wound healing. On reflection, rating down the strength of this evidence by a couple of levels from high to low because of the indirectness of the *outcome* would seem appropriate.

Are there situations where the strength of evidence can be justifiably raised after initially assigning a low level? Consider a systematic review of observational studies on the protective effect of bicycle helmets, compared to not wearing such helmets (cochranelibrary. com/cdsr/doi/10.1002/14651858.CD001855). This demonstrated a strong protective effect against head injury, a critical *outcome*. The overall effect size measured by summary odds ratio or OR was 0.31 with a 95% confidence interval of 0.26–0.37, indicating that the odds of head injury while cycling were reduced by two-thirds with the use of helmets compared to without them. At the outset, the level of strength of evidence is considered low due to the risk of bias in the observational study design. The bias may inflate the protective effect of the helmet observed in the review. However, it is unlikely that the large observed effect is solely due to the bias inherent in the observational design. The collated individual effects were taken from four studies that reported adjusted odds ratios accounting for confounding. The 'true' effect may be smaller, but it is unlikely that there would be no protective effect at all in reality. This raised our confidence in the observed effect and we have a good reason for rating up the level of strength of evidence from low to moderate.

Take, as another example, antibiotic treatment in otitis media (Box 5.2). The review found a reasonably large point estimate of effect. The summary relative risk point estimate was 0.37 for the critical *outcome* perforation of the eardrum, indicating that the odds of perforation under antibiotics were reduced by half. However, the 95% confidence interval around this point estimate ranged from 0.18 to 0.76, including the

Heterogeneity is the variation of effects between studies. It may arise because of differences in key characteristics of their *participants, interventions* and *outcomes* (clinical heterogeneity), or their study *designs* and quality (methodological heterogeneity).

Confounding is a situation in comparative studies where the effect of an *exposure* on an *outcome* is distorted due to the association of the *outcome* with another factor, which can prevent or cause the *outcome* independent of the *exposure*. Data analysis may be adjusted for confounding using multivariable models in observational studies.

Odds ratio (OR) is an effect measure for binary data. It is the ratio of odds in the experimental group to the odds in the control group. An OR of 1 indicates no difference between comparison groups.

Relative risk (RR) is an effect measure for binary data. It is the ratio of risk in the experimental group to the risk in the control group. An RR of 1 indicates no difference between comparison groups.

Box 5.2 Summary of results in a review of the effectiveness of antibiotics in otitis media among children

Importance of outcome	Outcome	Relative risk [95% CI]	Baseline risk (risk without treatment)	Risk under treatment* [95% CI]	Risk difference [95% CI]	NNT or NNH+ [95% CI]
Important	**Pain 2–3 days** 7 Trials (2320 participants)	0.70 [0.57–0.86]	159 per 1000 (16%)	111 per 1000 [90–137]	52 less per 1000 treated [22–69]	NNT: 20 [14–50]
Critical	**Perforation of eardrum** (assessed with otoscopy or examination of discharging ear within 7 days follow–up) 5 Trials (1075 participants)	0.37 [0.18–0.76]	47 per 1000 (5%)	17 per 1000 [8–36]	30 less per 1000 treated [11–39]	NNT: 33 [25–90]
Important	**Adverse effects** (Vomiting, diarrhoea, rash) 8 Trials (2107 participants)	1.38 [1.19–1.59]	196 per 1000 (20%)	270 per 1000 [233–311]	134 more per 1000 treated [37–115]	NNH: 14 [9–26]

Based on cochranelibrary.com/cdsr/doi/10.1002/14651858.CD000219.pub4.

* Risk under treatment is based on the risk without treatment and the odds ratio of the intervention is calculated using GRADEpro software freely available at gradeworkinggroup.org

+ NNT is the number needed to treat; NNH is the number needed to harm; see Box 5.4 for NNT computation.

possibility of a benefit as large as a reduction in odds by 82%. However, at the other extreme the confidence interval included a lower possibility of benefit at a 24% reduction in the risk of perforation under antibiotics. In yet another example, the confidence interval of the effect of anti-oestrogens as an infertility treatment crossed the line of no effect, i.e. RR = 1.0 (Box 4.4). This result leaves uncertainty about the true effect. We may, justifiably, make a judgment that this imprecision in the result merits lowering the level of strength of the evidence by a couple of levels, from high to low.

A dose–response relationship (sometimes also called biological gradient) would demonstrate that at higher doses the strength of association is increased. This can raise the level of strength of evidence from observational studies. Consider observational studies in Case study 9 which shows that rising body mass index increases prostate cancer mortality (Box C9.4). It is needless to say that criteria for raising and relegating the strength level of the evidence should be applied judiciously and transparently.

A **dose–response relationship** demonstrates that at higher doses the strength of association between exposure and outcome is increased.

5.2 Tabulating findings to aid interpretation

To improve transparency, a summary of findings' table should be prepared. The results and levels of strength of evidence should be stratified according to the *outcomes*. The number of studies and participants should be included per outcome to illustrate how much the body of evidence varies. The impact of antibiotic therapy in otitis media is investigated by seven studies with 2320 participants for the *outcome* pain on days 2–3, while five studies with 1075 participants assessed the prevention of perforation of the eardrum (Box 5.2).

The strength of the evidence should be evaluated separately for each *outcome*. This is because the strength of the evidence may vary across *outcomes*, even when the evidence comes from the same studies. For example, in the otitis media example (Box 5.3), take the outcome pain at 2–3 days. The strength of the evidence is high because the *participants*, *interventions* and *outcomes* refer directly to the question posed and there are no limitations in the methodological quality of the studies. The results are consistent across studies, the confidence interval around the point estimate of effect is narrow and there is no indication of publication bias. Similarly, the evidence strength level is also high for the *outcome* perforation of the eardrum. Case study 7 shows an example of relegating the strength level of evidence where there is a limitation in study quality (Box C7.4). In keeping our goal of reporting with transparency, whenever we decide to relegate or raise the strength level of the evidence for an *outcome*, it is important to report our judgments and reasons explicitly, using footnotes liberally in evidence tables.

Box 5.3 Assessing the strength of the evidence collated in a review of the effectiveness of antibiotics in otitis media among children

Outcome and its importance	Study design	Directness of outcome measure	Study quality (risk of bias)	Inconsistency of results (heterogeneity)	Imprecision of effects*	Publication bias	Strength of evidence†
Pain 2–3 days (Important)	Randomized trial *Initially assigned a high strength level*	Direct → *No change*	No limitations → *No change*	Consistent → *No change*	Precise → *No change*	Not detected → *No change*	*High*
Perforation of eardrum (Critical)	Randomized trial *Initially assigned a high strength level*	Direct → *No change*	No limitations → *No Change*	Consistent → *No change*	Precise → *No change*	Not assessed → *No change*	*High*
Adverse effects (Important)	Randomized trial *Initially assigned a high strength level*	Direct → *No change*	No limitations → *No Change*	Consistent → *No change*	Precise → *No change*	Not assessed → *No change*	*High*

Based on cochranelibrary.com/cdsr/doi/10.1002/14651858.CD000219.pub4.

* See Box 5.2 for confidence intervals of summary effects.

† See Box 5.1 for details.

5.3 Applicability of findings

By this time we must be thinking that we have reached the end. We already know if we can have sufficient trust in the review and we also have a good idea of the magnitude and range of the expected benefits (or harms or other outcomes). However, we need to do a bit more work before the applicability of the findings can be assessed.

We have measured the effects in relative terms (e.g. relative risk [RR] and odds ratio [OR]) as suggested in Box 4.2. Although the relative effect measures are useful for assessing the strength of the effect (and to perform meta-analysis), to judge whether an intervention is worthwhile, the absolute magnitude of the benefits, tailored to specific participant groups, is needed. This allows the clinical significance and the possible impact of the intervention to be understood. The absolute effect might be expressed as the risk difference (RD), which is a fraction, not a whole number (it is sometimes also called absolute risk reduction or ARR). The average human brain can only interpret natural frequencies or whole numbers well. The reciprocal of RD converts a fraction into a whole number called the number needed to treat (NNT). When dealing with an adverse effect, the same calculation is called the number needed to harm (NNH). However, this simple approach is only useful in dealing with data from individual studies. When using relative summary effect estimates obtained from reviews, the computation of the NNT is a bit more complicated and freely available software helps with calculation. This is explained in Box 5.4, but first we examine some virtues of NNTs.

Decision-making in healthcare is influenced by many factors. The size of the effect and its statistical significance in a meta-analysis provide only part of the information required. For example, when we interpret the summary effect, having received information about our patient's risk of an outcome without treatment, we might decide not to use it in low-risk patients as in our judgement the treatment associated morbidity and costs may not be worth the benefits. Thus, we may only use the treatment for patients at high risk. Relative effect measures tend to be constant across varying baseline risks, so they are not as informative when tailoring treatment decisions. The NNT, however, is sensitive to changing baseline risks and it allows us to individualize the benefit of interventions. The higher the NNT, the greater the number of patients clinicians must treat to achieve a beneficial effect in one patient. Therefore, they would be less inclined to recommend treatment and their patients would be more inclined to avoid treatment. Very often, in patients at higher baseline risk (i.e. worse prognosis), the NNT will be lower than in patients at lower risk (i.e. good prognosis). The lower the NNT, the smaller the number of patients clinicians must treat to achieve a beneficial result in one person; the more inclined a clinician would be to recommend treatment and the more enthusiastic their patients would be to have treatment.

Applicability (external validity or generalizability) is the extent to which the effects observed in a review can be expected to apply in routine clinical practice, i.e. to people who did not participate in the study.

Risk difference (RD) is an effect measure for binary data. In a comparative study, it is the difference in event rates between two groups. It is sometimes also called absolute risk reduction (ARR).

Number needed to treat (NNT) is the inverse of RD in individual studies. It is interpreted as how many participants would need to be treated to have one additional case of benefit.

Baseline risk is the risk or rate of *outcome* in a *participant* group without *intervention* (control group). It is related to the severity of the underlying disease and prognostic factors. Baseline risk is important for determining how many patients will likely benefit from an *intervention*.

Prognosis is a probable course or outcome of a disease. Prognostic factors are patient or disease characteristics which influence the *outcome*. A good prognosis is associated with a low rate of undesirable outcomes. Poor prognosis is associated with a high rate of undesirable outcomes.

How are NNTs generated from relative summary effects provided by reviews? A precondition is that the relative effects are in fact consistent across studies with varying baseline risks. Empirical evidence suggests that summary RR and ORs from meta-analysis using a random effects model are reasonably constant across various baseline risks. We can explore this phenomenon in our review by subgroup meta-analysis of studies stratified according to the prognostic category of the recruited patients. When such an analysis shows consistency in relative effects, we may use them to generate NNTs. We will of course need information on our patient's clinical condition and prognosis, which may require us to draw on evidence outside our effectiveness review. We might find that the evidence of the review moderated by the patient's specific circumstances might lead to different applications in different patients.

Box 5.4 Applying summary effects from reviews to clinical scenarios

Free-form question: Does aspirin in early pregnancy prevent the later onset of hypertensive disorders?

Structured question

• The participants	Women in early pregnancy
• The interventions	Low-dose aspirin
	Comparator: Placebo or no treatment
• The outcomes	Hypertensive disorders of pregnancy
• The study design	Experimental studies (*see Box 1.4*)

Summary of evidence of effectiveness of aspirin (Based on *BMJ* 2001; **322**: 329–33)

There were 32 relevant studies. Aspirin prevented hypertensive disorders of pregnancy with a summary relative risk (RR) of 0.85 (95% confidence interval 0.78–0.92). (RR values < 1.0 indicate an advantage for aspirin treatment compared to control.)

Exploring variation in relative effects of aspirin among various risk groups

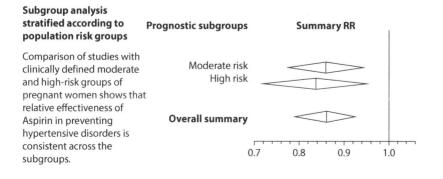

Individualizing aspirin prevention among various risk groups in early pregnancy

The number of women needed to be treated (NNT) with aspirin to prevent hypertension in pregnancy may be computed for various risk groups defined according to the clinical history and the results of the Doppler ultrasound test. This would aid in decision-making as one would be quite inclined to treat Doppler-positive women and not so inclined to treat Doppler-negative women according to the following NNTs.

Risk group	Baseline risk*	NNT+
Clinical history: High risk		
Doppler-positive	23.5%	29
Doppler-negative	7.8%	86
Clinical history: Moderate risk		
Doppler-positive	18.8%	36
Doppler-negative	2.5%	267

* *Based on a review of diagnostic accuracy of the Doppler test in predicting pregnancy hypertension (BJOG 2000; **107**: 196–208, doi: 10.1111/j.1471-0528.2000.tb11690.x).*

+ *Computed using the following formula:*

$$NNT = 1/[BR \times (1 - RR)], \text{ where BR is baseline risk and RR is 0.85}$$

If the summary effect measure is the odds ratio (OR), then the following formula is required:

$$NNT = [(1 - BR) + (OR \times BR)]/[BR \times (1-OR) \times (1-BR)]$$

*Based on BMJ 2001; **322**: 329–33, doi: 10.1136/bmj.322.7282.329.*

For example, considering the variation in NNTs among the risk groups outlined in Box 5.4, we might decide to treat Doppler-positive women but not Doppler-negative women among the clinically moderate risk group.

We consider the implications of individualizing summary effects from reviews to clinical scenarios using our earlier example of antibiotic treatment in children with otitis media (Box 5.2). At an RR of 0.70, antibiotics (compared with no treatment) will reduce pain at 2–3 days among children at moderate risk of this symptom from 16% to 11%. This translates into 52 fewer children with pain per 1000 cases treated or an NNT of 20. This beneficial effect has to be balanced against the adverse effects that antibiotics can induce, such as vomiting, diarrhoea and rash (Box 5.2). Case study 7 shows the comparison of adverse effects of two medications for antihypertensive treatment (Box C7.3). Judicious interpretation of findings of systematic reviews in different contexts is required to reach sound resolutions of scenarios.

> An **adverse effect** is an undesirable and unintended harmful or unpleasant reaction resulting from an *intervention*.

5.4 Generating recommendations

The usefulness of a review can be greatly enhanced by providing evidence-based bottom line messages to healthcare practitioners. This is usually done by providing the inferences from the review's findings.

A typical systematic review article does this in the discussion section of the paper (Box C10.3). Reviewers usually do this without formally assigning strength levels to the evidence collated. However, clinical practice guidelines go much further; they do this by generating formal practice recommendations from the tabulated findings of the evidence collated in the reviews per *outcome*, balancing beneficial *versus* harmful effects. This approach should be used universally in clinical practice guidelines, though not all guidance documents follow this approach. In systematic reviews as well in guidelines, there is considerable scope for confusion when moving from evidence synthesis to recommendations. In this section, we straighten out some common misconceptions and give a brief outline of the key factors to consider when generating recommendations for practice.

Recommendations should convey a clear message and should be as simple as possible to follow in practice (Case study 8). To achieve this, guideline developers need to start with high-quality reviews. This is the starting point for the development of recommendations for action in healthcare. What we and other practitioners really want to know about recommendations is how credible they are. By credibility, most people mean the trustworthiness and the reliability of a message. The credibility of a recommendation depends only in part on the strength of evidence collated from the review. Guideline developers need to make additional judgments on issues such as those listed in Box 5.5. Credibility requires that all judgements involved in a recommendation are made explicit. The criteria outlined in Box 5.5 provide one approach to explicitness in classifying recommendations as strong and weak. Needless to say, strong and weak recommendations can be in favour of or against a healthcare intervention. For example, in Case study 8, there is a positive recommendation in favour of mammography and a negative recommendation against clinical breast examination for cancer screening.

When assigning a strong or weak grade to a recommendation, at least four key factors need to be taken into consideration (Box 5.5). First is the balance between desirable and undesirable effects of an *intervention*, between its benefits and harms (Case studies 7 and 8). The second factor is the overall strength of the evidence behind the effects. Strong evidence is much more likely to result in a strong recommendation than effects observed in studies of low or even very low level of evidence strength. The third factor is the values and preferences that patients relate to the intervention. Finally, the fourth factor that influences the grading of a recommendation refers to the resource use that results from a recommendation, in particular (but not exclusively) cost. Although all recommendations have implications for resource use, many guidelines omit an explicit consideration of this factor in their decision. Low-cost effective interventions can be more easily afforded and transparency about how costs affect recommendations is an important feature of clinical practice guidelines.

Evidence-based medicine (EBM) is the conscientious, explicit and judicious use of current best evidence in making decisions about healthcare.

Clinical practice guidelines or just **Guidelines** are systematically developed statements that include recommendations to assist practitioners and patients in making decisions about specific clinical situations. Ideally, they should use evidence from **systematic reviews** with an assessment of the benefits and harms of alternative care options.

Box 5.5 Key considerations when generating recommendations

Considerations

1. **Balance between desirable and undesirable effects** (see Case studies 7 and 8)

   A large difference between desirable and undesirable effects increases the chances of a strong recommendation. A small difference increases the likelihood of a weak recommendation.

2. **Overall strength of evidence across all critical outcomes** (see Box 5.1)

   The higher the level of strength of the evidence, the higher the likelihood of a strong recommendation.

3. **Values and preferences**

   Large variations in values and preferences, or great uncertainty in values and preferences, increase the likelihood of a weak recommendation.

4. **Costs (resource allocation)**

   The higher the costs of an intervention, the lower the likelihood of a strong recommendation.

The implications of strong and weak recommendations

Implications	Strong recommendation	Weak recommendation
...for patients	Most patients in this situation would want the recommended course of action and only a small proportion would not.	Most people in this situation would want the recommended course of action, but many would not.
... for clinicians	Most patients should receive the recommended course of action.	Different choices will be appropriate for different patients, and the clinician must help each patient to arrive at a management decision consistent with the patient's values and preferences.
... for policymakers	The recommendation can be adopted as a policy in most situations.	Policy making will require substantial debate and the involvement of many stakeholders.

Recommendations are used by different groups such as healthcare professionals, patients and the general public, and local, regional or national policymakers. A strong or weak recommendation is likely to have different implications for each type of user. Healthcare professionals may interpret a strong recommendation as a directive advising them that almost all patients should receive the suggested action, and they may advise their patients accordingly. For patients, a strong recommendation may indicate that, when fully informed, most are very likely to make the same choice. Healthcare policymakers and funders may conclude from a strong recommendation that compliance with the suggested action could serve as a quality indicator to measure the performance of the organizations they commission to provide services.

A weak recommendation, on the other hand, may imply to clinicians that patients may vary in their values and preferences and as a result may take different courses of action despite the same evidence. In this situation, clinicians may therefore advise their patients to select a treatment that best suits their personal values. For patients, a weak recommendation may imply that a considerable proportion of patients would differ in their treatment choices. They might want to clarify their own preferences in this situation. Health policymakers may conclude from weak recommendations that compliance with suggested action will not be suitable as a quality indicator. In this scenario, a documented discussion with the patient on alternative treatment options would be a better standard of care criterion.

In summary, Step 5 provided guidance on how to take all the information from question framing to meta-analysis (Steps 1 to 4) into account when gauging the strength of the evidence in a systematic review and how to incorporate this into the process of making recommendations. A formal guideline document would tabulate the evaluations of evidence strength when making recommendations. A typical systematic review article would deploy what is outlined here to generate judicious inferences provided in the form of a narrative in the discussion section; the text size restrictions placed by journals usually would not permit detailed tabulation.

Writing tips for systematic review authors

- A typical systematic review paper is not expected to produce formal recommendations in the same way as guidelines do. The latter requires extensive documentation, and their reports usually far exceed in length than that of a standard peer-reviewed article. The tip here is that reviewers should decide early on in the writing process if they will present evidence grading tables, NNTs, etc. They would also need to decide if these should be included in the methods and results or just as interpretive information narrated in the discussion section.
- **Abstract:** Give the conclusion based on the strength of the evidence synthesized for the main critical outcome(s). If your chosen journal asks you to give the limitations under a specific subheading, the approach to evidence strength level evaluation in this Step will provide you with all the information needed.
- **Methods:** Ensure that the critical and important outcomes defined in the review question are underpinned by formal patient involvement or well-developed core outcomes set. If the paper is to formally report in the results section the strength of the evidence collated, the data synthesis subsection should provide the criteria used for raising or relegating strength levels. If the paper is to formally report the

IMRaD is an acronym that refers to the section headings used in writing the main manuscript text, i.e. I-Introduction, M-Methods, R-Results, a-and, D-Discussion, of a systematic review paper for submission to a peer-reviewed journal. See Case study 10 for tips, tricks and unwritten rules for convincing journal editors and peer-reviewers to publish your article.

individualization of the summary effects, the data sources for baseline risks used for calculating numbers needed to treat or harm should be identified.

- **Results:** Report the findings per outcome to permit evaluation of the strength of evidence per outcome having prespecified those that are critical and important. For each outcome, be sure to give study designs and quality (risk of bias), individual and overall effect estimates, 95% confidence intervals, I^2 statistics and funnel asymmetry statistics. The evidence strength tables can be provided as appendices. The reasons for raising or relegating the strength level of evidence should be detailed transparently in the footnotes of these tables. The tabulated information can be summarized diagrammatically as radar charts (Evid Based Med 2011;16:65-9, doi: 10.1136/ebm0005).

- **Discussion:** Give the conclusion based on the salience of the review's findings objectively interpreting the strength of evidence focusing on the main critical and important outcomes. Evidence for other outcomes should be considered as secondary findings. Comment on the role of patient and public involvement in determining the importance of outcomes. Make clear specific recommendations both for practice and research, whether or not formal strength of evidence evaluation is deployed. Recommendations for practice should emerge from consideration of the balance between desirable and undesirable effects of intervention, and the strength of evidence for each. If making recommendations for practice is unfeasible, simply stating that more research is needed is valueless unless specific study designs and methodologies are identified for use in future studies.

Summary of Step 5: Interpreting the findings

Key points about appraising review articles

- Are data on all critical and important outcomes reported?
- What is the level of strength of the evidence for each outcome?
- If the evidence in the review is trustworthy, what is its meaning for clinical practice?
- Are the authors' recommendations judicious?
- The article may not provide much of the analysis required for recommendations, but following the advice given in this Step, we might be able to generate clinically meaningful inferences for ourselves.

Key points about conducting reviews

- Specify the critical and important outcomes and set out the main findings for each separately.
- Ascertain that the key points about appraising and conducting reviews listed at the end of each of the four Steps so far have been met.

- Provide clinically meaningful inferences that emerge directly from the review's findings narratively even when formal evidence strength tabulation is not carried out.
- Assign a level of strength to the evidence for each outcome considering at least study design, methodological quality, consistency of results from study to study, the precision of observed effect and risk of publication and related biases.
- Explore variations in the relative effects and their reasons, particularly if the relative effects vary with baseline risk level or severity of the disease. The intervention may be effective only in certain clinical groups.
- Compute the predicted absolute effects (numbers needed to treat, NNTs) according to disease severity. This way we will be able to individualize the effects observed in the review to the requirements of patients.
- Any formal recommendations should be graded strong or weak considering the balance between desirable and undesirable effects, the strength of evidence across all critical and important outcomes, patients' values and preferences, and costs.

Section B: *Case studies*

The application of the review theory covered in the preceding section is illustrated through the following case studies. Some readers may prefer to assimilate the review theory first before turning to the case studies. Others may read them in conjunction with the information contained in the previous section. Each case consists of a scenario requiring evidence from reviews, a demonstration of some review methods and a proposed resolution of the scenario. The interpretations of the evidence are based on specific scenarios. Judicious interpretation of findings of systematic reviews in other scenarios may lead to different resolutions. Insight into critical appraisal and the conduct of a systematic review can be gained by working through the case studies.

Case study 1: Reviews of systematic reviews
Case study 2: Reviewing the safety of a public health intervention
Case study 3: Reviewing the effectiveness of therapy
Case study 4: Reviewing the accuracy of a test
Case study 5: Reviewing qualitative evidence to evaluate patient experience
Case study 6: Reviewing the effects of educational intervention
Case study 7: To use or not to use a therapy? Incorporating evidence on harmful outcomes
Case study 8: Review of clinical practice guidelines
Case study 9: Systematic reviews to assess a prognostic factor
Case study 10: Publishing systematic reviews: Tips and tricks for convincing journal editors and peer-reviewers

DOI: 10.1201/9781003220039-7

Case study 1: *Review of systematic reviews*

··

When seeking evidence from reviews to guide practice, we may face some difficulty as questions formulated in published reviews typically address the comparison of a single *intervention* or *exposure versus* control. This approach fails to take the broad clinical perspective; however, overviews of several reviews on a topic, called umbrella reviews, save the day. Such reviews frequently underpin practice guidelines and awareness about how to appraise them is important for evidence-based medicine.

This case study will demonstrate the advantages and disadvantages of umbrella reviews that cover broad questions. There are often various treatment options for a condition. How to appraise the findings of existing, frequently narrowly focused, reviews of these individual treatment options when they are combined within an umbrella review can be a challenge. This case study will help develop an approach to evaluating reviews which combines several reviews available on a topic. It will draw on the key points about appraisal (shown at the end of each Step in Section A) to make our reading of umbrella reviews more efficient.

Scenario: Preventing fractures in the elderly

You are a manager in a care home for the elderly where a resident has recently suffered a hip fracture. You have heard that vitamin D supplementation, with or without calcium, may be useful in prevention. You are due to attend a multidisciplinary case conference where you wish to put forward the possibility of using it for avoiding such morbidity among residents in the future. You have been thinking about examining the literature to check whether the best evidence backs your hunch or not.

Step 1: Framing the question

Free-form question

For adults in residential care homes, what is the effectiveness of the various vitamin D supplementation regimens for preventing fractures?

What is involved in conducting an umbrella review?
Framing questions
↓
Identifying relevant reviews
↓
Assessing the quality of the reviews included and their evidence
↓
Summarizing the evidence
↓
Interpreting the finding

An **umbrella review** is an evidence synthesis in the form of an overview of systematic reviews on a topic. Following a critical appraisal of all the relevant reviews, it might provide underpinning evidence for evidence-based practice or it might conclude that there is a need for conducting a new review. Where sufficient evidence is available for all alternative treatment options, it may be used to generate guidelines.

Effectiveness is the extent to which an *intervention* produces beneficial *outcomes* under ordinary day-to-day circumstances.

Structured question

The participants   Adults in residential care homes.
The interventions   Vitamin D supplementation, with or without calcium.
The outcomes   Prevention of hip fractures.
The study design   Systematic review(s) of experimental studies
                        addressing effectiveness.

The question formulated above is a broad one. Of the various components of the question, the *participant* description is quite focused, and the *interventions* and *outcomes* are broad. Vitamin D supplementation is the *intervention* to be considered, both alone and in combination with calcium. You wish to focus on a critical outcome, bone fractures, not just on intermediate outcomes. You expect to find a number of reviews, which would have taken a narrower focus, e.g. comparing vitamin D alone or vitamin D combined with calcium *versus* placebo. You want to choose prevention for your future residents with the optimum performance. For this, a sound umbrella review would likely provide the ideal evidence base.

Step 2: Identifying relevant reviews

The number of reviews has increased exponentially in recent years. When searching for reviews to guide your practice, you may be faced with numerous reviews collating the findings of several studies on your topic of interest. At first sight, this might fill you with enthusiasm. The reality is that multiplicity of reviews presents a challenge. Individual reviews may have a narrow focus on a single intervention. They may vary in currency and quality. Identifying which reviews to read and which not to may not be easy.

Search for reviews

From the sources of reviews shown in Box 0.1, you see that there are online repositories, such as KSR Evidence and Epistemonikos, exclusively for a systematic review, which can be searched. General databases like PubMed also permit searches to be limited to systematic reviews. Having framed your question, you decide to search PubMed. It is a key source of reviews with 216,519 relevant citations in 2021, at the time of writing.

There are several ways to find reviews in PubMed. Just by typing the words 'vitamin D supplementation' AND 'hip fractures' in the query box, clicking the search button and limiting the search to systematic reviews, there are 31 hits (11 in the last 5 years). Adding the words 'umbrella review' to the above search reduced the number of hits to 1; yes, one only. You decide that this review of systematic reviews is suitable for addressing your question:

● Vitamin D supplementation and fractures in adults: A systematic umbrella review of meta-analyses of controlled trials. *J Clin Endocrinol Metab* 2022; **107**: 882–98, doi: 10.1210/clinem/dgab742.

Free-form question:
It describes the query for which you seek an answer through a review in simple language (however vague).

Structured question:
Reviewers convert free-form questions into a clear and explicit format using a structured approach (see Box 1.2). This makes the query potentially answerable through existing relevant studies.

Question components
The participants:
A clinically suitable sample of patients.

The interventions:
Comparison of groups with and without the intervention.

The outcomes:
Changes in health status due to interventions.

The study design:
Ways of conducting research to assess the effects of interventions.

Effect is a measure of association between an *intervention* and an *outcome*.

Box C1.1 Searching PubMed for umbrella reviews on vitamin D supplementation for preventing hip fractures

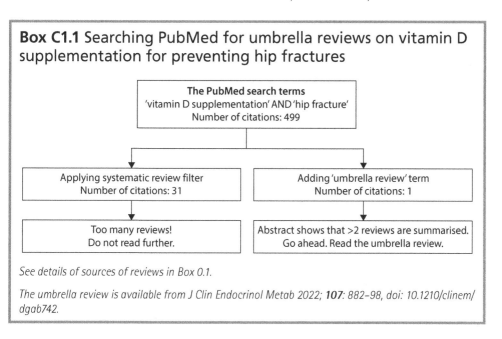

The PubMed search terms
'vitamin D supplementation' AND 'hip fracture'
Number of citations: 499

Applying systematic review filter
Number of citations: 31

Adding 'umbrella review' term
Number of citations: 1

Too many reviews!
Do not read further.

Abstract shows that >2 reviews are summarised.
Go ahead. Read the umbrella review.

See details of sources of reviews in Box 0.1.

*The umbrella review is available from J Clin Endocrinol Metab 2022; **107**: 882–98, doi: 10.1210/clinem/ dgab742.*

Step 3: Assessing the quality of the included reviews

The umbrella review overviewed several individual systematic reviews, each with its own methods. A two-step approach is required for the assessment of quality in this situation. First, an assessment of the overall quality of the umbrella review is required. This is facilitated by the use of key points about review appraisal at the end of each Step in Section A of this book. Next, an assessment of the quality of the individual reviews included in the umbrella review is required. One cannot just accept the findings of the collated reviews without a quality appraisal. For convenience within an umbrella review and standardization across reviews, one of the published systematic review quality assessment checklists can be deployed.

Having reassured yourself that the umbrella review is overall of reasonable quality, you turn to the individual included reviews (Box C1.2). In this umbrella review, the AMSTAR-2 checklist was applied to assess the quality of the included reviews (Box C1.3). Taking a closer look at the amount and quality of the evidence included in each of the reviews when interpreting the findings, this checklist assesses confidence in the results of the review as being: high, if there is no critical weakness and no more than one non-critical weakness; moderate, if there is no critical weakness

AMSTAR-2: The second version of AMSTAR (A MeaSurement Tool to Assess systematic Reviews), an instrument for evaluating the quality of systematic reviews (amstar.ca).

ROBIS: An instrument for assessing the Risk Of Bias In Systematic reviews (bristol.ac.uk/ population-health-sciences/projects/ robis/robis-tool).

Box C1.2 Appraising the overall quality of a review of systematic reviews of vitamin D supplementation for the prevention of hip fractures

Step 1: Framing questions

- The overview was based on predefined questions with prospective registration.
- The questions seem not to have been modified during the review.

Step 2: Identifying relevant literature

- The searches appear to be comprehensive.
- The selection criteria were set *a priori* and applied by multiple reviewers independently.
- It seems unlikely that relevant reviews might have been missed.

Step 3: Assessing the quality of the literature

- Quality assessment has been undertaken for the included reviews.
- Quality has been used as a criterion for selection (Step 2): Effectiveness assessment reviews of experimental studies were included.
- A more detailed quality assessment of selected reviews has been carried out using the AMSTAR-2 tool (Box C1.3). The quality items are appropriate for the question.
- Variation in quality has been explored as an explanation for heterogeneity (Step 4).

Step 4: Summarizing the evidence

- Overlap of primary studies within included reviews has been formally assessed.
- Heterogeneity of effects within included reviews has been evaluated.
- The exploration for heterogeneity was planned within reported subgroup analyses in the included reviews.
- Variation in primary studies' clinical characteristics has not been found to be an explanation for heterogeneity.
- Variation in primary studies' quality has not been found to be an explanation for heterogeneity.
- Meta-analysis was used by individual reviews included but not in the umbrella review data synthesis.

Step 5: Interpreting the findings

- Risk of publication and related biases has not been formally addressed in the umbrella review (no method exists for this at the time of writing) and it has been addressed in a limited way in the included reviews.
- The conclusions are focused on a critical outcome and are clearly made with consideration of the quality of the included reviews.
- The strength of the evidence included in the umbrella review has not been graded; the grading is high within the moderate-quality included review.

- The umbrella review's findings provide recommendations to generate inferences for practice.

A critical appraisal based on key points is listed at the end of each step in Section A of this book.

The umbrella review is available from J Clin Endocrinol Metab 2022; 107: 882–98, doi: 10.1210/clinem/dgab742.

and more than one non-critical weaknesses; low, if there is one critical weakness with or without non-critical weaknesses; and critically low, if there is more than one critical weakness with or without non-critical weaknesses. Of the individual reviews included concerning the effect of vitamin D supplementation alone without calcium on hip fractures, only one has moderate quality. Similarly, of the individual reviews included concerning the effect of vitamin D supplementation with calcium on hip fractures, only one has moderate quality.

Box C1.3 Assessing the quality of included individual systematic reviews within an umbrella review using the AMSTAR-2 checklist

Confidence in the findings of an included individual systematic review	Weaknesses		Included systematic reviews on the effect of vitamin D supplementation with calcium *versus* placebo on hip fractures
	Critical items*	Non-critical	
High – moderate	0	1–2	1
Low	1	+/–	1
Very low	≥2	+/–	10

AMSTAR-2 checklist items modified from original (critical items marked with an asterisk): Structured questions and inclusion criteria including question components; *Prospective registration and justification of any deviations from the protocol; Explanation of study designs for inclusion; *A comprehensive literature search; Study selection and data extraction in duplicate; *Listing excluded study justification; Description of included studies in detail; *Assessment of study quality for the risk of bias; *Appropriate use of meta-analysis; *Evaluation of the impact of quality in evidence synthesis and interpretation; Seeking an explanation for heterogeneity; *Investigation of publication and related biases; and Reporting sources of funding for the studies included, and the reviewers' own conflict of interest.

AMSTAR-2 is available from amstar.ca.

ROBIS, another instrument for assessing the risk of bias in systematic reviews, is available from bristol.ac.uk/population-health-sciences/projects/robis/robis-tool.

The umbrella review is available from J Clin Endocrinol Metab 2022; 107: 882–98, doi: 10.1210/clinem/dgab742.

Step 4: Summarizing the evidence

The umbrella review had 19 systematic reviews comparing vitamin D supplementation alone *versus* placebo/control and 13 systematic reviews on vitamin D supplementation with calcium *versus* placebo/control. The question was formulated to compare vitamin D supplementation alone *versus* vitamin D in combination with calcium. They are each compared to placebo in head-to-head comparisons in the reviews included. Using placebo/control as a common comparator, it is possible to indirectly compare vitamin D supplementation alone *versus* vitamin D in combination with calcium.

There is no effect of vitamin D supplementation alone *versus* placebo/control on hip fractures. There is an effect of vitamin D supplementation with calcium *versus* placebo/control on reduction in hip fractures, underpinned by the moderate quality individual reviews included. Eight of 12 reviews evaluating the *outcome* hip fracture reported a significant reduction in risk; the summary relative risk was 0.84 (95% confidence interval 0.74–0.96, without heterogeneity I^2 0%) in the moderate-quality included review. This effect is seen specifically within the subgroups of studies concerning institutionalized and elderly adults.

Step 5: Interpreting the findings

It is important to assess the strength of evidence when interpreting the findings using the key points from Step 5. The available evidence for the effectiveness of vitamin D supplementation with calcium was, in general, of low or very low quality. The evidence strength within the moderate-quality review included in the umbrella review is high. With this moderate-quality systematic review concerning the critical *outcome* hip fracture, you are reassured that the preventive benefit of vitamin D supplementation with calcium merits consideration, but vitamin D alone should be discarded as an option.

Resolution of scenario

Having considered the evidence yourself, you are more confident about your proposal for hip fracture prevention in your residential home. You decide to take the umbrella review to the multidisciplinary case conference and make a short presentation about the strength of the evidence for discussion. The input of the key stakeholders present at this meeting will help to determine an evidence-based residential home fracture prevention policy where vitamin D supplementation with calcium will be included along with other good practices.

Strength of evidence describes the extent to which we can be confident that the estimate of an observed effect is correct for important outcomes. It takes into account the directness of outcome measure, study design, study quality (risk of bias), heterogeneity, imprecision of the effect (confidence interval width) and publication bias (this is not an exhaustive list).

Network meta-analysis is an advanced meta-analytic technique that may be used in umbrella reviews addressing broad questions comparing multiple *interventions* for the treatment of the same condition. The details of this technique are not covered in this book.

Case study 2: *Reviewing the safety of a public health intervention*

Reviews of the safety of interventions are not as common as those of their effectiveness. Research on safety may relate to common harmful outcomes, which may be captured in the same studies that address effectiveness. However, most experimental studies focus primarily on effectiveness and secondarily on safety – any information on safety is often only a by-product. Harmful outcomes can be rare and they may develop over a long time. There are considerable difficulties in designing and conducting safety studies to capture these outcomes, as a large number of people need to be observed over a long period of time. In this situation, observational, not experimental, studies are needed. With this background, systematic reviews on safety have to include evidence from studies with a range of designs.

This Case study demonstrates how to seek and assess evidence on safety using a published review of a preventive public health intervention. This topic is important because public health interventions have an impact on large groups of people and it has to be assured that the benefit outweighs any potential harm. This Case study provides a demonstration of the application of review theory related to question formulation, literature identification and quality assessment of studies on safety. It was developed as a learning aid in 2002. For the third edition of this book, we searched the literature for reviews published since the year 2000. There were not many new citations concerning reviews of drinking water fluoridation. The question of its safety appeared to have been addressed by only a few citations and settled by the 2000 systematic review incorporated in the original Case study 2. So we decided to keep this Case study on safety in a form close to how it was presented in the first edition.

Step 1 Framing questions
↓
Step 2 Identifying relevant literature
↓
Step 3 Assessing the quality of the literature
↓
Step 4 Summarizing the evidence
↓
Step 5 Interpreting the findings

Safety relates to adverse effects associated with *interventions*.

Effectiveness is the extent to which an *intervention* produces beneficial *outcomes* under ordinary day-to-day circumstances.

Scenario: Safety of public water fluoridation

You are a public health professional in a locality that has public water fluoridation. For many years, you and your colleagues have held the belief that it improves dental health. Recently your local authority has been under pressure from various interest groups to consider the safety of this public health intervention because they fear that it is causing cancer.

In the past, most public health decisions have been based on judgement and practical feasibility; however, in recent years there has been

DOI: 10.1201/9781003220039-9

an increasing demand to examine the scientific basis behind the issues under consideration. You have been observing this development with interest and now you have the chance to apply this approach yourself. In anticipation of the discussion about the safety of water fluoridation intensifying in the near future, you want to prepare well and use evidence from the literature to inform any future decisions.

Having framed your question, you search PubMed from the sources of reviews shown in Box 0.1. By typing the words 'water fluoridation' AND 'safety' in the query box and clicking the search button, there are 151 hits. Although you are a bit shocked about this large number of studies and are wondering how to squeeze the necessary reading time into your already packed daily routine, you apply the Systematic review filter in the above PubMed search. You find seven citations. Reading through titles and abstracts, you decide that the following review is suitable for addressing your question:

- Systematic review of water fluoridation. *BMJ* 2000; **321**: 855–9, doi: 10.1136/bmj.321.7265.855

Incidentally, if you do an Internet search on the same day using the Google search engine (google.com), you will have an overwhelming 7,720,000 hits in under a second, but in the first position among them will be the above systematic review. There are several governmental reports but they all tend to rely on the paper you already found in PubMed. The full report of the systematic review on which this paper is based is also available:

- A systematic review of water fluoridation. NHS Centre for Reviews and Dissemination (CRD) Report 18. York, University of York, 2000 (york. ac.uk/inst/crd/fluorid.htm)

Your impression is that using the review is the right starting point as it may save an enormous amount of time compared with obtaining and reading a large number of individual studies.

Free-form question: It describes the query for which you seek an answer through a review in simple language (however vague).

Structured question: Reviewers convert free-form questions into a clear and explicit format using a structured approach (see Box 1.2). This makes the query potentially answerable through existing relevant studies.

Step 1: Framing the question

Free-form question

Is it safe to provide population-wide drinking water fluoridation to prevent caries?

Structured questions

The participants People receive drinking water sourced through a public water supply.

The exposures Fluoridation of drinking water (naturally or artificially) compared with non-fluoridated water.

The outcomes	Cancer is the main outcome of interest for the debate in your health authority. You also decide to consider other outcomes such as fluorosis (mottled teeth) and fractures as there has been a concern about the effect of fluorides on bones.	
The study designs	Comparative studies of any design (Box 1.4) examining the outcomes in at least two participant groups, one with fluoridated drinking water and the other without.	

Question components

The participants:
A suitable sample of participants.

The exposures:
Comparison of groups with and without the exposure.

The outcomes:
Changes in health status due to interventions.

The study design:
Ways of conducting research to assess the effect of interventions.

The published review was conducted to address five different questions. This Case study will only focus (for the sake of brevity and simplicity) on the question of safety related to the *outcomes* described above.

Step 2: Identifying relevant literature

To cast as wide a net as possible to capture as many relevant citations as possible, a wide range of medical, political and environmental/scientific databases were searched to identify primary studies of the effects of water fluoridation (Box C2.1). The range of databases searched in this

---

Box C2.1 Identification of relevant literature on the safety of public water fluoridation

Electronic databases searched

1. Agricola
2. BIOSIS Previews (a database on life sciences)
3. CAB Health
4. CINAHL (Cumulative Index of Nursing and Allied Health Literature)
5. Conference Papers Index
6. EI Compendex (Engineering Index)
7. EMBASE (Excerpta Medica Database)
8. Enviroline
9. Food Science and Technology Abstracts (FSTA)
10. Health Service Technology, Administration and Research (Healthstar)
11. HSR Proj
12. JICST-E Plus (Japanese Science and Technology)
13. Latin American and Caribbean Health Sciences Literature (LILACS)
14. MEDLINE and OldMEDLINE
15. NTIS
16. PASCAL
17. PSYCLIT

18. Public Affairs Information Service (PAIS)
19. Science Citation Index and Social Science Citation Index
20. System for Information on Grey Literature in Europe (SIGLE)
21. TOXLINE
22. Water Resources Abstracts
23. Waternet

Study identification flow chart

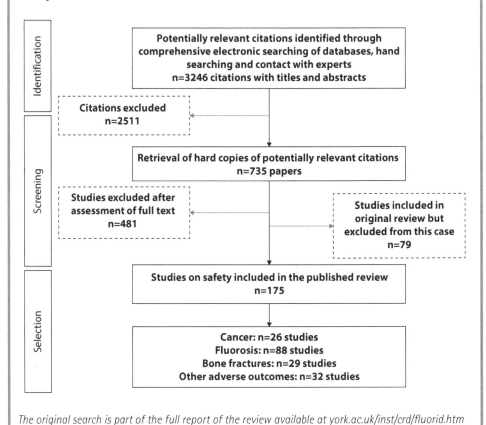

The original search is part of the full report of the review available at york.ac.uk/inst/crd/fluorid.htm

review is far beyond what is usually covered in reviews of clinical questions. The electronic searches are also supplemented by hand searching Index Medicus and Excerpta Medica for several years (back to 1945) to cover the time period before Medline and Embase became accessible electronically. The search process was further supported by the use of the Internet. Various Internet search engines were used to find web pages that might provide references. In addition, web pages were set up to inform the public about the review and to enable individuals and organizations to submit references or reports. Not surprisingly, there was a degree of duplication in the captured citations resulting from searching a wide range of databases. After the removal of duplicates, 3246 citations remained, from which the relevant studies were selected for review.

This comprehensive search of a variety of databases yielded far more citations than are commonly found when searching the literature for focused clinical questions (compare with Case study 3). The potential relevance of the identified citations was assessed – 2511 citations were found to be irrelevant. The full papers of the remaining 735 citations were assessed to select those primary studies in humans that directly related to fluoride in drinking water supplies, comparing at least two groups. These criteria excluded 481 studies, leaving 254 studies in the review. They came from 30 countries and were published in 14 languages between 1939 and 2000. Of these studies, 175 were relevant to the question of safety (Box C2.1).

Identifying relevant literature
- Develop search term combinations
- Search relevant electronic databases
- Search other relevant resources
- Obtain full papers of potentially relevant citations
- Include/exclude studies using preset selection criteria

Step 3: Assessing study quality

Study design threshold for study selection

The use of *study design* as a marker for ensuring a minimum level of quality has been described as an inclusion criterion in Step 2. This approach is easier to apply when seeking evidence of effectiveness using experimental studies. This is because randomized studies are often difficult (if not impossible) to conduct at a community level for a public health intervention such as water fluoridation. Thus, systematic reviews assessing the safety of such interventions have to look beyond experimental studies and include evidence from various types of *study design*. Considering the nature of the research likely to be available to address safety issues, in this review a simple *design* threshold was used as a selection criterion: Comparative studies of any design were included, but those without any comparative information were excluded (Box 2.4). In this way, studies that provided information about the harmful effects of exposure to fluoridated water compared with non-exposure were selected.

Confounding
is a situation in comparative studies where the effect of an *exposure* on an *outcome* is distorted due to the association of the *outcome* with another factor, which can prevent or cause the *outcome* independent of the *exposure* and it is also associated with the *exposure*. Data analysis may be adjusted for confounding in observational studies.

Quality assessment of safety studies

After selecting studies of an acceptable design, their in-depth assessment of the risk of various biases allows us to gauge the quality of the evidence in a more refined way. The objective of the included studies is to compare groups exposed to fluoridated drinking water with groups without such exposure and look for rates of undesirable outcomes without bias. Step 3 shows how to develop and use study quality assessments in a review of effectiveness. For safety studies to have validity, they must ascertain *exposures* and *outcomes* in such a way that the risk of misclassification is minimized. They must also establish the association between

A comparative study is one where the effect of an *exposure* is assessed using comparison groups.

exposures and *outcomes*, adjusting for the confounding effect of other factors. These features are likely to be more robustly implemented in experimental studies, but they typically assess a relatively small number of participants over a short duration of follow-up. So in such studies there is only a limited chance of detecting rare *outcomes* that often do not follow immediately after *exposure*. Hence, quality assessment has to be planned somewhat differently from that in reviews of the effectiveness of interventions. In this Case study, the quality issues related to safety studies are briefly examined.

Anticipating that experimental studies would be scarce, reviewers planned study quality assessments based on features that would minimize biases of the various types described above. They assessed ascertainment of *exposures* and *outcomes*, i.e. how did the investigators make sure that the study participants had the *exposures* and *outcomes* under question. A prospective design would facilitate this. This means that those exposed (and unexposed) to fluoridated water and those developing cancer (and remaining free of cancer) are more likely to be correctly identified in these groups if they are assessed in a prospective fashion. The *exposure* is likely to be more accurately ascertained if the study commenced soon after water fluoridation and the *outcomes* are likely to be more accurately ascertained if the follow-up is long and if it is assessed blind to *exposure* status.

When examining how the effect of *exposure* on *outcome* was established, reviewers assessed if the comparison groups were similar in all respects other than their exposure to fluoridated water. This is because the other differences may be related to the *outcomes* of interest independent of the drinking water fluoridation, and this would bias the comparison. For example, if the people exposed to fluoridated water had other risk factors that make them more prone to cancer, the apparent association between *exposure* and *outcome* may be explained by the more frequent occurrence of these factors among the exposed groups compared with the non-exposed groups. Technically speaking, such studies suffer from confounding. In a (large) experimental study, confounding factors are expected to be approximately equally distributed between groups (but no such studies exist on water fluoridation). In observational studies, their distribution may be unequal. Primary researchers can statistically adjust for these differences when estimating the effect of *exposure* on *outcomes* (using multivariable modelling). The larger the number of variables adjusted for, the more likely it is that the observed association between *exposure* and *outcome* will be 'true'.

Put simply, use of a prospective design, robust ascertainment of *exposure* and *outcomes*, and control for confounding are the generic issues one would look for in a quality assessment of studies on safety. Assessing these methodological features in safety studies of water fluoridation will require the development of quality criteria specific to this topic. For example, studies commencing within 1 year of water fluoridation would be able to ascertain *exposure* better than those commencing

The **validity** of a study depends on the degree to which its design, conduct and analysis minimize **biases**.

Bias either exaggerates or underestimates the 'true' effect of an *exposure*.

Effect is a measure of association between an *exposure* and an *outcome*.

within 1–3 years, which in turn will be better than those commencing after 3 years. This way studies would range from satisfactorily meeting quality criteria, to having some deficiencies, to not meeting the criteria at all, and they can be assigned to one of the three pre-specified quality categories as shown in Box C2.2.

Box C2.2 A quality assessment checklist for studies on the safety of public water fluoridation

Quality (risk of bias) assessment checklist

	Quality categories	
Quality items	High* – moderate	Low
Prospective design	Prospective	Prospective or retrospective
Exposure ascertainment	Study commenced within 3 years of water fluoridation	Study commenced after 3 years of water fluoridation
Outcome ascertainment	Long follow-up and blind assessment	Short follow-up and unblinded assessment
Control for confounding	Adjustment for at least one confounding factor	No adjustment for confounding factors

* *High-quality studies were prospective, commencing within 1 year of water fluoridation, followed up people for at least 5 years, used blinding (or other robust methods) to ascertain outcomes and adjusted for at least three confounding factors (or used randomization) – no such studies existed.*

Description of study quality (risk of bias) assessment

Information on quality is presented as 100% stacked bars separately for studies evaluating different harmful outcomes. Data in the stacks represent the number of studies in moderate- and low-quality categories. There were no high-quality studies.

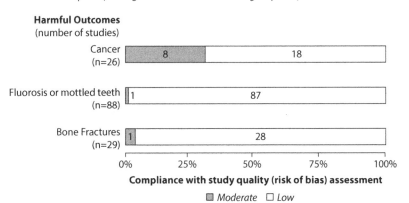

The Newcastle-Ottawa Scale (NOS), an instrument that standardizes the quality assessment of observational studies included in a systematic review, provides a generic checklist covering the concepts described in this box (ohri.ca/programs/clinical_epidemiology/oxford.asp).

Description of quality of the selected studies

Based on the degree to which studies comply with the quality criteria, a quality hierarchy can be developed (Box C2.2). None of the included studies is in the highest quality category, but this is because experimental studies are non-existent and control for confounding is not always ideal in observational studies (none is adjusted for three or more confounding factors in the analysis). Many studies lacked a prospective design, which makes ascertainment of *exposure* and assessment of *outcomes* difficult. More details of the study quality may be obtained from the review, but the general dearth of quality evidence in reviews of the safety of interventions is not surprising to those experienced in this field.

The quality assessment for studies addressing the three harmful *outcomes* assigns low quality to the vast majority of the available evidence; only a few studies are classified as having medium quality, and none has high quality (Box C2.2). Fortunately (because cancer is of major interest in this Case study) studies examining the association between fluoridation and cancer show the highest quality as compared to those examining the other two harmful *outcomes* related to bones.

Step 4: Summarizing the evidence

Summarizing the evidence from studies with a large variety of designs and quality is not easy as highlighted in Steps 4 and 5. The review provides details of how the differences between study results were investigated and how they were summarized (with or without meta-analysis). This Case study restricts itself to summarizing the findings narratively for the outcomes discussed below.

Cancer

The association between exposure to fluoridated water and cancer in general was examined in 26 studies. Of these, 10 examined all-cause cancer incidence or mortality in 22 analyses. Eleven analyses found a negative association (fewer cancers due to exposure), nine found a positive association and two found no association. Only two studies found statistical significance. Thus, no clear association between water fluoridation and increased incidence or mortality was apparent. While a broad number of cancer types were represented in the included studies, bone/joint and thyroid cancers were of particular concern due to fluoride uptake by these organs. Six studies of osteosarcoma and water fluoridation reporting variance data found no statistically significant differences. Thyroid cancer was considered by only two studies and these also did not find a statistically significant association with water fluoride levels. Overall, from the research evidence presented, no association was detected between water fluoridation and mortality from any cancer or from bone or thyroid cancers specifically. These findings were also borne out in the moderate quality subgroup of studies.

Fluorosis

Dental fluorosis is the most frequently studied harmful outcome, as reflected by the largest number (88) of studies included. Meta-regression analysis showed a strong (statistically significant) association between the fluoride level and the prevalence of dental fluorosis.

Bone fractures

Twenty-nine of the included studies investigated a variety of fracture sites; hip fracture was included in 18 of them. There are no definite patterns of association for any of the fractures. Similarly to the cancer studies, the studies showed similar numbers of positive and negative associations. Hip fracture analysed as a subgroup also showed no association with exposure to fluoridated drinking water.

Step 5: Interpreting the findings

In this case scenario, you focused on the safety of a community-based public health intervention. The generally low quality of available studies means that interpretation must be with appropriate caution. The elaborate efforts in searching an unusually large number of databases provide some safeguard against missing relevant studies and ongoing research. The strength of the evidence summarized in this review is likely to be low, but it is as good as it is going to get in the foreseeable future.

Cancer is the *outcome* of most interest in the case scenario. No association is found between *exposure* to fluoridated water and specific cancers or all cancers. The interpretation of the results in this review may be limited because of the low quality of studies, but the findings for the cancer *outcomes* are also supported by moderate quality studies.

Fluorosis (mottled teeth) shows a simple association and also a dose-response relationship with increasing exposure to water fluoridation. When compared with a fluoride level of 0.4 ppm (parts per million), a level of 1.0 ppm had an estimated number needed to treat (NNT) of 6 (range 4–21), sometimes called the number needed to harm (NNH) in this context. This means that, on average, for every six people exposed to the higher concentrations of fluorides, one additional person has mottled teeth. Bone fractures did not show an association with water fluoridation.

> The **strength of the evidence** lies in the relevance of the outcomes, the methodological quality of the included studies, the heterogeneity of results, the precision and size of effects, etc., features that underpin the trust in the inferences generated from a review.

> A dose–response relationship demonstrates that at higher doses the strength of association between exposure and outcome is increased.

Resolution of the scenario

After having spent some time reading and understanding the review, you are impressed by the sheer amount of literature relevant to the question of safety. However, you are somewhat disappointed about the poor quality of the available primary studies. Of course, examining safety only makes sense in a context where the intervention has some beneficial effect. Benefit and harm have to be compared to provide the basis for decision-making. Regarding the issue of the beneficial effect of public water fluoridation, you are reassured by the review that your prior belief and that of your health authority are correct: drinking water fluoridation does prevent caries. You can now go on to evaluate the findings of the review on safety – reduction in caries by introducing fluoridation can be considered in context with cancer, fluorosis, bone fractures and other problems.

When the pressure from the interest groups raises the profile of the safety issue again, you will be able to reassure them that there is evidence to demonstrate that drinking water fluoridation is not linked to cancer. You will also be able to reassure them that there is no risk of fractures to bones. However, you will have to admit the risk of dental fluorosis, which appears to be dose dependent. Those concerned about this issue can be given advice about examining their fluoride intake from other means. You may also want to measure the fluoride concentration in your area's water supply to openly share this information with the interest groups.

Being able to quantify the safety concerns of your population through a review, albeit from studies of moderate–low quality, allows your health authority, politicians and the public to consider the balance between beneficial and adverse effects of water fluoridation. For some, the prevention of caries is of primary importance, so they would prefer fluoridation. On the other hand, aesthetic reasons may play a more important role for others who would prefer to have caries removed occasionally rather than have mottled teeth. In any case, you are able to reassure all parties that there is currently no evidence of a risk of cancer or bone fractures from drinking water fluoridation.

Case study 3: *Reviewing the effectiveness of therapy*

Step 1
Framing questions
↓
Step 2
Identifying relevant literature
↓
Step 3
Assessing the quality of the literature
↓
Step 4
Summarizing the evidence
↓
Step 5
Interpreting the findings

Not all reviews can provide answers that have immediate practical implications. And this may be due to a dearth of relevant studies. But the scarcity of evidence of effectiveness should not be interpreted as evidence of lack of effectiveness.

This Case study will demonstrate how to seek and assess evidence of therapeutic effectiveness in a review and how to act when faced with limited evidence. Based on a published review, it will provide a good demonstration of the application of review theory related to literature identification, study quality assessment and data synthesis without meta-analysis. It was developed as a learning aid in 2002. For the third edition of this book, we searched the literature for reviews published since the year 2000. The question of antimicrobial therapy for chronic wounds appeared to have been addressed by only a few citations and the 2000 systematic review incorporated in the original Case study 3 remains a comprehensive evidence synthesis suitable for teaching and learning. So we decided to keep this Case study on effectiveness in a form close to how it was presented in the first edition.

Scenario: Antimicrobial therapy for chronic wounds

You are a clinical research fellow in an academic primary healthcare practice. There are a large number of patients with chronic wounds of various aetiologies. You have taken it upon yourself to develop an evidence-based clinical strategy for use of antimicrobials in the management of these patients. Your initial discussions with other members of the practice reveal that they base their management on:

- what they had learnt many years ago during medical school,
- what they observed from the nurses on the wards during postgraduate training, and
- what they have been told by pharmaceutical company representatives.

Hardly anybody could underpin their advice with good evidence. There are a variety of antimicrobial products and there seems to be no clear way forward.

You are keen to conduct a review yourself but, sensibly, you first decide to see if there is one already out there in the literature. Having framed your question, you search PubMed from the sources of reviews shown in Box 0.1. Typing the words 'chronic wounds' AND 'antimicrobial' in the query box and clicking the search button, there are 4757 hits.

You imagine that this large number of studies must have been summarized in a review, so you apply the Systematic review filter in the above PubMed search. You find 60 citations. Reading through titles and abstracts on the first page sorted by best match, you decide that the following review is suitable for addressing your question:

- Systematic review of antimicrobial agents used for chronic wounds. *Br J Surgery* 2001; **88**: 4–21, doi: 10.1046/j.1365-2168.2001.01631.x

You also search the Cochrane Library, looking at other sources of review given in Box 0.1, and find no current, relevant review to directly address your question. Incidentally, if you did an Internet search on the same day using the Google search engine (google.com), you will have an overwhelming 35,200,000 hits in under a second, but in the first position among them will be the above systematic review. You decide the read this review in detail to gain the knowledge summarized.

Step 1: Framing the question

Free-form question

Which of the many available antimicrobial products improve healing in patients with chronic wounds?

Structured question (also see Boxes 1.2 and 1.3)

The participants	Adults with various forms of chronic wounds are being cared for in an ambulatory setting. We narrow down the definition of chronic wounds to diabetic ulcer, venous ulcer, pressure ulcer and chronic ulcer (excluding pilonidal sinus – which was included in the related reviews – from further consideration in this Case study).
The interventions	Systemic or topical antimicrobial preparations (e.g. antibiotics, antifungal, antiviral, antiseptic agents) compared with usual treatment, placebo or alternative antimicrobial products (excluding studies about prevention).
The outcomes	A range of assessments for wound healing, e.g. complete healing, change in ulcer size, rate of healing, time to heal, etc. Complete wound healing is the clinically relevant outcome while the rest are surrogates.
The study designs	Comparative studies with or without randomization (selection of non-randomized studies restricted to those with a concurrent control group).

Question components

The participants: A clinically suitable sample of patients.

The interventions: Comparison of groups with and without the intervention.

The outcomes: Changes in health status due to interventions.

The study design: Ways of conducting research to assess the effect of interventions.

Clinically relevant *outcomes* directly measure what is critical and important to patients in terms of how they feel, what their function is and whether they survive.

Surrogate *outcome* **measurements** substitute for direct outcome measures. They include physiological variables or measures of subclinical disease. To be valid, the surrogate must be correlated with the clinically relevant outcome.

Core *outcomes* are a group of critical and important outcomes on which there is consensus that they should be measured and reported. Systematic reviews are used to create a long list of outcomes which is then reduced to a core outcomes set through surveys collating evaluations of patients and practitioners.

Step 2: Identifying relevant literature

A comprehensive search was undertaken by the reviewers (without language restrictions) to identify as many relevant published and unpublished studies as possible. The electronic search covered 17 databases from their inception to January 2000 (Box C3.1). The combination of search terms used for the Medline database is shown in Box C3.2. Other databases were searched using a modified combination of these terms. In addition, manual searches of five relevant journals not covered by the electronic databases, 12 proceedings of relevant meetings and bibliographies of all retrieved articles were undertaken. A panel of subject experts was also consulted to identify studies not captured by the searches. Examples of going to such great lengths to hunt down relevant literature are not as common as one might think in the field of systematic reviews. The initial search provides 400 possibly relevant citations. After screening their titles and abstracts, 150 papers are retrieved for examination of the full text. Despite the exhaustive efforts, ultimately only 22 studies (including over 1000 patients) are found that address the question posed.

Identifying relevant literature
- Develop search term combinations
- Search relevant electronic databases
- Search other relevant resources
- Select citations to retrieve potentially relevant papers
- Include/exclude studies using preset selection criteria

Box C3.1 Identification of relevant literature on antimicrobials for chronic wounds

Electronic databases searched*

1. BIOSIS Previews (a database on life sciences)
2. British Diabetic Association Database
3. CINAHL (Cumulative Index of Nursing and Allied Health Literature)
4. CISCOM (Centralised Information Service for Complementary Medicine)
5. Cochrane Database of Systematic Reviews (CDSR)
6. Cochrane Wounds Groups developing database
7. Current Research in Britain (CRIB)
8. Database of Abstracts of Reviews of Effectiveness (DARE)
9. DHSS (Database produced by the Department of Health, UK on health services provided by the NHS nursing and primary care; people with disabilities and elderly people)
10. Dissertation Abstracts
11. EMBASE (Excerpta Medica Database)
12. Index to Scientific and Technological Proceedings
13. ISI® Science Citation Index
14. MEDLINE (*see search term combinations in Box C3.2*)
15. National Research Register (NRR)
16. Royal College of Nursing Database
17. System for Information on Grey Literature in Europe (SIGLE)

Study identification flow chart

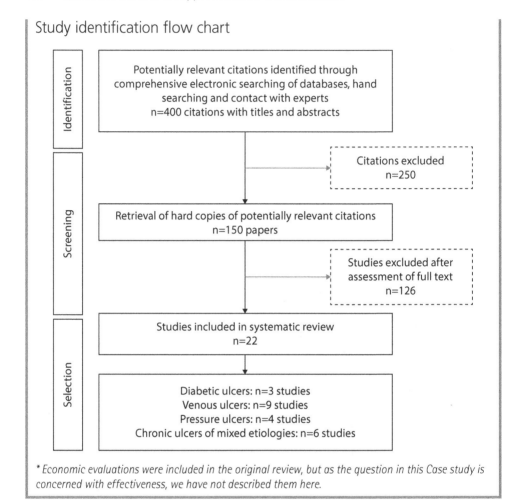

Identification

Potentially relevant citations identified through comprehensive electronic searching of databases, hand searching and contact with experts
n=400 citations with titles and abstracts

Citations excluded
n=250

Screening

Retrieval of hard copies of potentially relevant citations
n=150 papers

Studies excluded after assessment of full text
n=126

Selection

Studies included in systematic review
n=22

Diabetic ulcers: n=3 studies
Venous ulcers: n=9 studies
Pressure ulcers: n=4 studies
Chronic ulcers of mixed etiologies: n=6 studies

* Economic evaluations were included in the original review, but as the question in this Case study is concerned with effectiveness, we have not described them here.

Step 3: Assessing study quality

Study design threshold for study selection

From the outset, there was a worry that only a few studies with sound designs would be available. So the threshold for study selection had been lowered to allow observational studies with concurrent controls to be included along with randomized controlled trials and experimental studies without randomization (Box 1.4). Comparative studies with historical controls and case-control studies were excluded because of the higher risk of bias associated with these designs (Box 2.4). Of the 22 studies selected, 18 claimed to be experimental studies (but only four were clearly randomized, though with some deficiencies in the concealment of allocation), and four were observational cohort studies with concurrent controls.

Study design filter employs a search term combination to capture citations of studies of a particular design.

Box C3.2 Search term combination for Ovid Medline database to identify citations on antimicrobials for chronic wounds

The original search term combination consists of 58 sets of terms. The following table shows only a selection of these. The purpose is to demonstrate how to build a search term combination.

Question components and a selection of relevant terms	Type of terms		Boolean operator (see glossary)
	Free	MeSH	
The participants: Patients with various forms of chronic wounds			
1. decubitus ulcer/ or foot ulcer		x	
2. leg ulcer/ or varicose ulcer/		x	
3. skin ulcer/		x	
4. diabetic foot/		x	
5. ((plantar or diabetic or heel or venous or stasis or arterial) adj. ulcer).tw	x		OR (captures *participants*)
6. ((decubitus or foot or diabetic or ischaemic or pressure) adj. ulcer).tw	x		
7. (pressure or bed) adj. Sore$	x		
8. *additional terms (see in original report of the review)*			
9. or/1–9			
The interventions: Treatments for chronic wounds			
10. debridement/ or biological dressings/ or bandages		x	
11. occlusive dressings/ or clothing/ or wound healing/		x	
12. antibiotics/ or growth substances/ or platelet derived growth factor/		x	
13. (debridement or dressing$ or compress$ or cream$ or (growth adj factor$)).tw	x		OR (captures *intervention*)
14. antibiotic$ or (electric adj therapy) or laser$ or nutrition$ or surg$).tw	x		
15. (homeopath$ or acupuncture or massage or reflexology or ultrasound).tw	x		
16. *additional terms (see in original report of the review)*			
17. or/10–17			

The outcomes
No search is performed to capture *outcomes*

| 18. and/9,17 | | | AND (combines *participants* and *intervention*) |

| Question components and a selection of | Type of terms | | Boolean operator |
relevant terms	Free	MeSH	*(see glossary)*
The study designs			
19. random allocation/ or randomized controlled trials/		x	
20. controlled clinical trials/ or clinical trials phase I/ or clinical trials phase II/		x	
21. single-blind method/ or double blind method/		x	OR (captures *study designs*)
22. ((random$ adj controlled adj trial$) or (prospective adj random$).tw.	x		
23. *additional terms (see in original report of the review)*			
24. or/19–23			
18 and 24			AND (combines *participants* and *intervention* and *study designs*)
25. limit 25 to human			

Commands and symbols for Ovid Medline

$ Truncation, e.g. antibiotic$ will pick up antibiotics in general as well as different types of antibiotics (e.g. antibiotics, aminoglycosides; antibiotics, lactam)

adj   Proximity and adjacency searching, e.g. chronic adj wounds$ means that these terms appear next to each other

.tw   Textword search, e.g. skin adj ulcer.tw will search for these adjacent textwords in title or abstract

/   Medical subject heading (MeSH) search, e.g. diabetic foot/ will search for MeSH in indexing terms

The original search is part of the full report of the review available at journalslibrary.nihr.ac.uk/hta/hta4210#/full-report

Description of quality (risk of bias) of the selected studies

The development of a quality (risk of bias) checklist is outlined in Box C3.2. The selected studies are systematically examined for key generic biases: Is there potential for selection bias? For performance bias? For measurement bias? Or for attrition bias? (Box 3.2). At the same time, quality issues specific to the *participants*, *interventions* and *outcomes* of the review question were considered. In this review, the appropriateness of inclusion and exclusion criteria and comparability of groups at baseline for the severity of ulcers was particularly important because there were concerns about the inadequacies of methods used for minimizing selection bias. Assessment of the wound healing process to determine *outcomes*

Bias either exaggerates or underestimates the 'true' effect of an *intervention*.

The **quality** of a study depends on the degree to which its design, conduct and analysis minimize **biases**.

is critical even when measurement bias is minimized by blinding *outcome* assessors. This is because *outcome* assessment could be qualitatively different. For example, when assessing healing, the *outcomes* could be any one of complete healing, ulcer healing quotient, healing index, improvement scores, etc. Complete healing should be regarded as the most important *outcome* due to its importance to patients. Considering both generic and specific issues, a quality (risk of bias) checklist with a total of nine items can be developed as shown in Box C3.3.

This checklist is applied to studies included in the review (Box C3.4), but the quality is often unclear due to a lack of reporting. Where information on quality is available, many studies fall short of meeting the desired quality. For example, even when studies purport to be randomized, there are deficiencies both in sequence generation and in allocation concealment.

Box C3.3 A quality assessment checklist for studies on the effectiveness of antimicrobials for chronic wounds

The clinical question and selection criteria

- Nature of question   Assessment of effectiveness
- Study design   Evaluation of the effectiveness of therapy, focusing on how one treatment compares with another (*see Box 1.4*)
- Study design threshold   Inclusion criteria: Randomized controlled trials
      Experimental studies without randomization
      Cohort studies with concurrent controls
      Exclusion criteria: Studies with historical controls
      Case-control studies

The study quality (risk of bias) assessment checklist

a) Generic quality items for a checklist (see also Boxes 3.2 **and** 3.3**)**

- **Adequate generation of random sequence for allocating patients to interventions**
  Computer generated random numbers or random numbers tables
- **Adequate concealment of allocation**
  Robust methods to prevent foreknowledge of the allocation sequence to clinicians and patients, e.g. centralized real-time or pharmacy-controlled randomization in unblinded studies, or serially numbered identical containers in blinded studies
- **Adequate blinding**
  Care provider, study patients and outcome assessors
- ***A priori* sample size estimation**
- **Description of withdrawals**
  Numbers and reasons provided for each group
- **Intention-to-treat analysis** (ITT)
  Inclusion of all those who dropped out/were lost to follow-up in the analysis so that the calculations indeed follow the ITT principle

b) Specific quality items related to clinical features of the review question

- The participants
  Correct inclusion/exclusion criteria
  Comparison of severity of wound condition at baseline
- The interventions
  No items
- The outcome
  Importance of outcomes: Complete healing (critical); ulcer healing quotient, healing index, improvement scores and microbial growth (surrogates)

See Box C3.4 for a description of study quality.

ROB-2, the second version of the Cochrane Risk Of Bias instrument for assessing the quality of randomized trials (methods.cochrane.org/risk-bias-2), and ROBINS-I, an instrument for assessing the Risk Of Bias In Non-randomised Studies of Interventions (methods.cochrane.org/methods-cochrane/robins-i-tool), provide generic checklists covering the concepts described in this box.

Box C3.4 Description of the quality (risk of bias) assessment of studies on antimicrobials for chronic wounds

Quality items

Quality item	Yes	Unclearly reported	No
Adequate random sequence generation	4	17	1
Adequate allocation concealment	1	17	4
Adequate blinding	10	5	7
A priori sample size estimation	2	20	
Intention-to-treat analysis	6	6	10
Description of withdrawals	10	7	5
Correct inclusion/exclusion criteria	16	.	6
Baseline comparison	14	6	2
Outcome: Complete wound healing	14	7	

Compliance with quality items (0% – 100%)

■ Yes ☐ Unclearly reported ☐ No

Information on quality is presented as 100% stacked bars. Data in the stacks represent the number of studies.

See Box C3.3 for related information on quality items.

Step 4: Summarizing the evidence

A brief descriptive summary of the studies' characteristics and effects is tabulated in Box C3.5. A number of treatment comparisons were available but only in studies with a small number of patients (range 8–52 per group). Duration of follow-up also varied (range 2–20 weeks) and there was no consistency in measures of *outcomes*. This variation in what is done to whom, over what period and how *outcomes* are assessed introduces clinical heterogeneity and this makes a meaningful synthesis of results difficult (and makes meta-analysis impossible).

An examination of the observed effects in individual studies shows large values for point estimates of odds ratios (OR), but most effects are not statistically significant as the 95% confidence intervals (CI) include the possibility of no beneficial effect or even a harmful effect. For example, Wunderlich (1991) found that a silver-based product SIAX was better than various control regimens with an OR of 3.9 but the 95% CI is 0.7–22.1. Similarly, Alinovi (1986) showed that the healing rate was worse when standard care was supplemented by systemic antibiotics compared with standard care alone with an OR of 0.54, but 95% CI is 0.1–1.9. Even when effects were statistically significant, e.g. Morias (1979) reports OR 20.3 (95% CI 1.1–375.1), the estimation is quite imprecise due to the small sample size. Considering the low quality of the studies, one could hardly be enthused to trust such a result, even when it is statistically significant.

Step 5: Interpreting the findings

This review shows that research on the value of different antimicrobial products in wound care is scarce. Despite an exhaustive search effort, there are only a few relevant studies (Box C3.1) and their quality is relatively low (Box C3.4). A descriptive summary of the evidence shows that the observed effects are seemingly good (perhaps one reason why these studies are published despite their low quality), but they are imprecise, as insufficient numbers of patients are studied (Box C3.5). Technically speaking, the studies are likely to be underpowered. In this situation, the studies are unable to detect an effect when one possibly exists, so one cannot prove the lack of effectiveness of the *interventions*. None of the numerous antimicrobials currently in use for various types of chronic ulcers has been robustly assessed, i.e. with appropriate design and conduct, clinically relevant *outcomes* and a large enough sample size. Thus, no recommendations can be made regarding the superiority or lack of effectiveness of any of the antimicrobial agents. Needless to say, additional research is needed in the form of well-designed randomized controlled trials.

Resolution of the scenario

You are taken by surprise by the quantity and quality of the body of evidence on such a common problem as chronic wounds, which have a significant impact on healthcare resources in your primary healthcare setting.

Effect is a measure of association between an *intervention* and an *outcome*.

Point estimate of effect is its observed value in a study.

Confidence interval is the imprecision in the point estimate, i.e. the range around it within which the 'true' value of the effect can be expected to lie with a given degree of certainty (95%). This reflects uncertainty due to the play of chance.

Heterogeneity is the variation of effects between studies. It may arise because of differences between studies in key characteristics of their *participants, interventions* and *outcomes* (clinical heterogeneity), and their *study designs* and quality (methodological heterogeneity).

Power is the ability of a study to statistically demonstrate an effect when one exists. It is related to sample size and the number of outcomes in the comparison groups. The larger the sample size, the more the power, and the lower the risk that a possible effect could be missed due to the play of chance.

Box C3.5 A brief summary of the findings of studies included in a systematic review on antimicrobials for chronic wounds

(not all comparisons included in the original review are presented in this table)

Participant subgroups	Interventions (number of patients/ulcers in the group)		Outcomes		Effects
Study author and year of publication	Control group (standard/placebo)	Experimental group	Observation period	Outcome measure[+]	Effect estimate[*] (95% CI)
Diabetic ulcer					
Systemic treatments					
Chanteleau 1996	Placebo (22)	Antibiotics (22)	3 weeks	Complete healing	OR: 0.45 (0.1–1.6)
Lipsky 1990	Cephalexin (29)	Clindamycin (27)	2 weeks	Complete healing	OR: 1.31 (0.4–4.0)
Topical treatments					
Vandeputte (unpublished)	Hydrogel (15)	Chlorhexidine (14)	12 weeks	Complete healing	OR: 0.07 (0.007–0.7)
Venous ulcer					
Systemic treatments					
Huovinen 1994	Ciprofloxacin (12)	Trimethoprim (12)	12 weeks	Complete healing	OR: 2.14 (0.38–12.2)
Alinovi 1986	Standard (24)	Antibiotics + standard (24)	3 weeks	Complete healing	OR: 0.54 (0.1–1.9)
Topical treatments					
Pierard-Franchimont 1997	Hydrocolloid (21)	Povidone iodine + hydrocolloid (21)	8 weeks	Median healing index	ES: 1.00 (−0.4–2.4)
Bishop 1992	Placebo (29)	Silver sulphadiazine (30)	4 weeks	Complete healing	OR: 7.57 (0.8–67.4)
Cameron 1991	Non-medicated tulle gras (15)	Mupirocin-impregnated tulle gras (15)	12 weeks	Complete healing	OR: 1.31 (0.31–5.49)
Salim 1991	Allopurinol (51)	Dimethyl sulphoxide (50)	12 weeks	Complete healing	OR: 2.04 (0.36–11.69)
Wunderlich 1991	Various preparations (20)	Silver impregnated activated charcoal dressing (20)	6 weeks	Complete healing	OR: 3.86 (0.7–22.1)
Blair 1988	Saline (30)	Silver sulphadiazine (30)	12 weeks	Complete healing	OR: 0.43 (0.14–1.38)
Pegum 1968	Lint (17)	Polynaxylin + lint (17)	Until healed	Mean ulcer healing quotient	ES: −0.30 mm²/day (−2.1–1.5)

Pressure ulcers

Topical treatments

Study	Control treatment	Experimental treatment	Duration	Outcome measure	Effect estimate
Della Marchina 1997	Alternative spray (10)	Antiseptic spray (9)	15 days	Complete healing	OR: 2.57 (0.19–34.6)
Toba 1997	Povidone iodine/sugar (11)	Gentian violet 0.1% blended with dibutyryl cAMP (8)	14 weeks	Mean % base-line ulcer area remaining	ES: 11.1 (−8.69–30.89)
Gerding 1992	A&D ointment (13)	DermaMend (26)	4 weeks	No. of improved scores	OR: 6.57 (1.30–33.34)
Huchon 1992	Hydrocolloid (38)	Povidone iodine (38)	8 weeks	Improved scores	OR: 0.46 (0.2–1.4)
Chronic ulcers of mixed aetiology					
Systemic treatments					
Valtonen 1989	Disinfectant (8)	Ciprofloxacin + disinfectant (18)	12 weeks	Complete healing	OR: 3.84 (0.2–83.5)
Morias 1979	Placebo (29)	Levamisole (30)	20 weeks	Complete healing	OR: 20.33 (1.1–375.1)
Topical treatments					
Worsley 1991	Hydrocolloid (12)	Povidone iodine ointment (15)	12 weeks	Complete healing	OR: 0.31 (0.05–2.08)
Beitner 1985	Saline (10)	Benzoyl peroxide 20% (10)	6 weeks	Mean % remaining ulcer area	ES: 34.10 (21.1–47.1)
Margraf 1977	Various agents (10)	Silver zinc allantoine cream (10)	Until healed	Mean days to heal	ES 59.0 (34.12–83.88)
Marzin 1982	Benzoyl peroxide (20)	Collagen gel (20)	12 weeks	Wound area remaining	No effect estimate reported ($p < 0.01$)

[+] In studies with several outcome measures, the most clinically important one is presented using the following hierarchy: complete healing > ulcer healing quotient, healing index, improvement scores > microbial growth.

[*] Odds ratio (OR) > 1 and effect size (ES) > 0 indicate improved outcome with experimental treatment.

See Box 4.1 for advice on construction of tables.

For you, it is currently not possible to inform a clinical policy on the management of chronic wounds with robust evidence.

Scarcity of evidence of effectiveness does not equate with evidence of lack of effectiveness! So you decide to form the most sensible policy using common sense and the consensus of your colleagues (this keeps everyone happy). However, you obtain an agreement to periodically seek new evidence and update your policy when new robust evidence becomes available.

To help fill the gap in evidence that you have identified through this review, there are some other options open to you. To help generate the new evidence:

- the least you can do is submit this topic to relevant research funding bodies for prioritization,
- you can also design and commence a robust systematic review update using the guidance in this book, and
- you can encourage colleagues to actively recruit patients in a relevant clinical trial if there is one ongoing.

Case study 4:
Reviewing the accuracy of a test

Step 1
Framing questions
↓
Step 2
Identifying relevant
literature
↓
Step 3
Assessing the quality
of the literature
↓
Step 4
Summarizing the
evidence
↓
Step 5
Interpreting the
findings

No document of approximately 2000 words, the size of this Case study, can purport to do justice to systematic reviews of test accuracy literature. We make no attempt to be comprehensive here as the virtually infinite number of methodological nuances in test accuracy research demand a textbook in this field.

In this Case study, we reinforce the general principles behind systematic reviews by demonstrating their application in a scenario concerning the use of evidence about the accuracy of a test. It provides a good demonstration of study quality assessment, quantitative synthesis and interpretation of findings.

Scenario: Ultrasound scan test for postmenopausal women with vaginal bleeding

You are a clinician responsible for women's health in a primary care centre serving a relatively large retired population. You are often faced with women who present with unexpected episodes of vaginal bleeding after menopause. You know that in the past these patients used to be routinely investigated by gynaecologists using uterine curettage under anaesthesia. This practice is now considered outdated, but the current local practice still involves referral to a specialist based in a tertiary care setting. You wonder if an ultrasound scan of the uterus can exclude pathology accurately in postmenopausal women with abnormal vaginal bleeding. In this way, women who test negative will not need a referral to tertiary care.

You search PubMed from the sources of reviews shown in Box 0.1 to see if there are any relevant reviews in the literature. You type 'ultrasound postmenopausal bleeding' in the query box and click the Go button. There are 1067 citations. You filter the results to focus on systematic reviews, ticking the Systematic Review checkbox on the left-hand side of your screen. There are now only 17 citations and on the first page the following seemingly relevant citation is staring at you:

- Ultrasound detection of endometrial cancer in women with post-menopausal bleeding: Systematic review and meta-analysis. *Gynecol Oncol* 2020; **157**: 624–33, doi: 10.1159/000520878.

Step 1: Framing the question

Free-form question

Among postmenopausal women with abnormal vaginal bleeding, does an ultrasound scan exclude uterine cancer accurately?

Structured question

The participants	Postmenopausal women in the community with symptoms of vaginal bleeding.
The index test	Endometrial thickness measurement during ultrasound imaging of the pelvis and the uterus (see Box C4.1). You are mainly interested in the accuracy of the negative test result.
The reference standard	Endometrial cancer is confirmed histologically. There are many abnormalities of the endometrium and the uterus (benign, pre-cancer and cancer). Endometrial cancer is the most important one. Focusing on this diagnosis is not unreasonable (not least for the sake of simplicity in this Case study). You are mainly interested in excluding the diagnosis of cancer.
The study design	Test accuracy study (Box C4.3), i.e. observational studies in which results of a test (endometrial ultrasound) are compared with the results of a reference standard (endometrial histology).

Step 2: Identifying relevant literature

An electronic search was carried out to capture all the relevant citations about ultrasound of the endometrium and then those citations were identified that evaluate ultrasound among postmenopausal women with vaginal bleeding to predict the likelihood of endometrial cancer. Medline database was searched using PubMed and the search was not restricted by language literature. The search term combination included MeSH and keywords of 'endometrial neoplasms' AND 'ultrasonography' AND 'metrorrhagia'. The electronic search was coupled with manual scanning of bibliographies of known primary and review articles to identify relevant papers (Box C4.2). In total, 44 studies (including 17,339 women) were included in the review. Of these, 20 studies (including 10,165 women)

Box C4.1 Ultrasound scan of the pelvis and the uterus

In ultrasound imaging of the uterus, the endometrium (lining of the womb) is described in terms of thickness and regularity. Regular endometrium of less than 5 mm thickness is often used to define a threshold or cut-off for abnormality. An example of a normal test result is shown below.

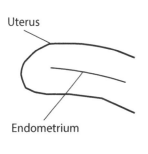
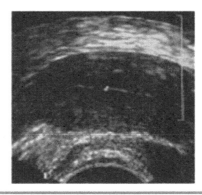

---

were on the accuracy of endometrial thickness, at the most frequently used 5 mm abnormality threshold, to predict the diagnosis of endometrial cancer.

MeSH or medical subject headings are controlled terms used in the Medline database to index citations. Other bibliographic databases use MeSH-like terms.

Step 3: Assessing study quality

Quality assessment of test accuracy studies

An accuracy study is different from an effectiveness study. It is designed to generate a comparison between measurements obtained by a test and those obtained by a reference standard. A reference standard is a test that confirms or refutes the presence or absence of disease beyond a reasonable doubt. Therefore, it is sometimes also known as the 'gold' standard. We shall give a basic explanation of the *design* of a test accuracy study (Box C4.3) and its quality features (Box C4.4)

There are many possible sources of bias in accuracy studies, as shown in Box C4.4. Selection bias may arise if the sample is not suitably representative of the population. This is less likely to occur when using consecutive or random sampling. Poor descriptions of *test* and *reference standards* in terms of preparation of the patients, details of measurements, computation of results and thresholds for defining abnormality are also associated with bias. The *reference standard* should be a recognized 'gold' standard and it should be administered independently of the *test*. In addition, observers assessing *reference standards* for verification of diagnosis should be kept blind to measurements obtained

The **quality** of a study depends on the degree to which its design, conduct and analysis minimize **biases**.

Bias either exaggerates or underestimates the 'true' accuracy of a test.

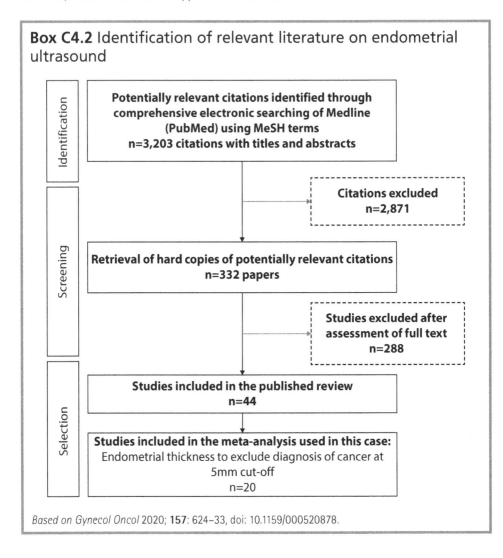

Box C4.2 Identification of relevant literature on endometrial ultrasound

Based on *Gynecol Oncol* 2020; **157**: 624–33, doi: 10.1159/000520878.

from the *test* and *vice versa*. Blinding avoids bias because recordings made by one observer are not influenced by the knowledge of the measurements obtained by other observers. During the verification process, bias may arise if the *reference standard* is not applied to all patients, or if it is differentially applied to test-positive and test-negative cases.

A detailed quality checklist was used for the assessment of test accuracy studies on endometrial ultrasound using the principles outlined in Step 3. The original version of QUADAS, a QUality Assessment tool for Diagnostic Accuracy Studies, was used to evaluate the risk of bias in the accuracy studies included in the review (Box C4.4). An overview of the relevant generic aspects of test accuracy studies in this review reveals that the ultrasound *test* and the histological examination of the

Box C4.3 Design of test accuracy studies evaluating endometrial ultrasound

Simple description of study design

An observational study that tests subjects from a relevant population and compares its results with those of a reference standard. For example, studies comparing results of endometrial ultrasound with those of endometrial histology in women with postmenopausal bleeding.

Study flow chart with key generic quality features

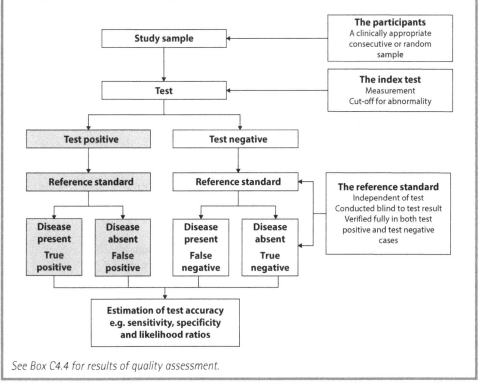

See Box C4.4 for results of quality assessment.

Box C4.4 Quality assessment of test accuracy studies evaluating endometrial ultrasound using the 14-item QUADAS tool*

- Was the spectrum of participants representative of the patients who will receive the test in practice?
- Were selection criteria clearly described?
- Is the reference standard likely to correctly classify the target condition?
- Is the time period between reference standard and index test short enough to be reasonably sure that the target condition did not change between the two tests?

- Did the whole sample or a random selection of the sample receive verification using a reference standard of diagnosis?
- Did patients receive the same reference standard regardless of the index test result?
- Was the reference standard independent of the index test?
- Was the execution of the index test described in sufficient detail to permit replication of the test?
- Was the execution of the reference standard described in sufficient detail to permit its replication?
- Were the index test results interpreted without knowledge of the results of the reference standard?
- Were the reference standard results interpreted without knowledge of the results of the index test?
- Were the same clinical data available when test results were interpreted as would be available when the test is used in practice?
- Were uninterpretable and intermediate test results reported?
- Were withdrawals from the study explained?*

The current version of the tool is named QUADAS-2 (see Glossary).

See Box C4.5 for a graphic presentation of selected quality items used for the assessment of studies included in this Case study.

endometrium, which serves as the *reference standard*, are independent. So, the remaining methodological issues related to recruitment of patients, blinding of observers and completeness of verification of diagnosis are examined.

Among quality issues related specifically to the review question, a sufficient description of the *participants* to demonstrate that the sample is representative of the disease spectrum seen in practice is essential, otherwise the estimates of accuracy may be biased. For the *test, a priori* setting of the 5 mm threshold is crucial, as post hoc determination of threshold is subject to manipulation in light of the findings of the study. Finally, for the *reference standard*, the use of adequate endometrial sampling is crucial to the validity of the selected studies. Adequate methods of obtaining endometrial samples include hysterectomy and directed biopsy.

Study design threshold for study selection

In this review, a quality threshold in study selection was used to exclude all studies with a case-control design. These studies would have selected cases with and without cancer and patients' records would be retrospectively examined if their endometrial ultrasound scans were abnormal. Such a design has been empirically shown to be associated with bias, leading to an exaggeration of test accuracy.

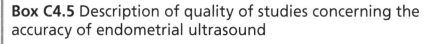

Box C4.5 Description of quality of studies concerning the accuracy of endometrial ultrasound

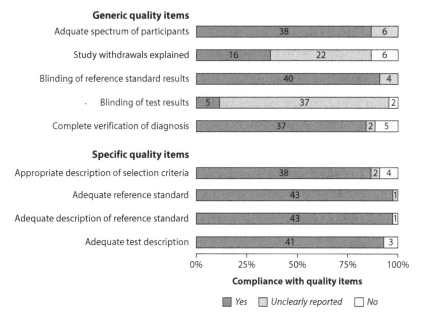

Information on quality is presented as 100% stacked bars. Data in the stacks represent the number of studies.

Based on Gynecol Oncol 2020; **157**: 624–33, doi: 10.1159/000520878.

See Box C4.4 for related information on the quality items.

Description of study quality for selected studies

Box C4.5 indicates the quality of 44 selected studies for a selection of the quality items taken from the QUADAS tool. For most of the quality items, the lack of compliance with good quality features was due to a lack of reporting. In general, there were deficiencies of one sort or another among all studies.

Step 4: Summarizing the evidence

This Case study describes the estimates of the accuracy of individual studies, the examination of heterogeneity of accuracy across studies and the meta-analysis of individual accuracy estimates among studies using 5 mm thickness as the threshold for abnormality (other details of included studies can be obtained from the original paper). But first we must understand how to choose a measure of accuracy (Box C4.6).

Likelihood ratio (LR) of a positive (or negative) test is the ratio of the probability of a positive (or negative) test result in subjects with a disease to the probability of the same test result in subjects without the disease. The LR indicates by how much a given test result will raise (if positive) or lower (if negative) the probability of having the disease.

Box C4.6 Estimation of accuracy in studies evaluating tests

Measures of test accuracy

These are statistics for summarizing the accuracy of a test. For binary tests, there are three commonly used pairs of accuracy measures: positive and negative predictive values; sensitivity and specificity; and likelihood ratios (LRs). Unlike measures of effect, single measures of accuracy are infrequently used.

Computing accuracy for binary test results

A way of computing accuracy measures is shown below. Predictive values give the probability of having a disease and not having a disease among subjects with positive and negative test results, respectively. Sensitivity and specificity give the probability of a positive and a negative test result among subjects with and without disease, respectively. Positive and negative LRs describe the probabilities of obtaining a test result (positive or negative) in subjects with the disease relative to individuals without the disease. However, to compute accuracy of several studies and to estimate its uncertainty (its confidence interval), manual calculations can become tedious. We suggest you use statistical software.

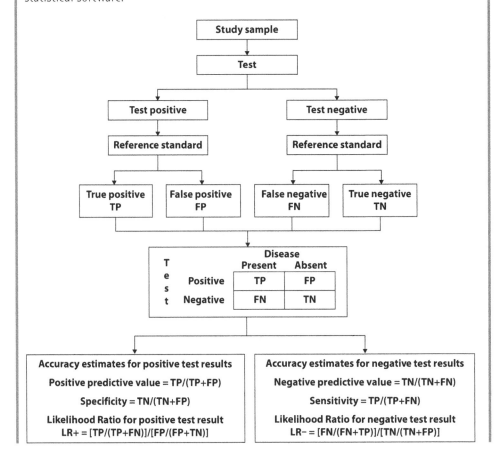

Choosing accuracy measures for binary tests

There is a debate about which measures are preferable and how best to pool them across several studies in a meta-analysis. No single approach is entirely satisfactory. LRs are more clinically meaningful because when they are used in conjunction with information on disease prevalence (pre-test probability), they help to generate post-test probabilities as shown in Box C4.8. Pooling of individual sensitivity (Sn) and specificity (Sp) results should take into account their interrelationship, as they may not behave independently. Bivariate method and summary ROC (receiver operating characteristics) plot allow for pooling of results from individual studies taking account of the relation between Sn and Sp. LRs are not suitable for pooling in the meta-analysis, particularly when the threshold for abnormality varies from study to study. The preference for LRs over other accuracy measures for clinical interpretation can be met by deriving these from Sn and Sp as LR+ = [Sn/(1 – Sp)] and LR– = [(1 – Sn)/Sp].

See relevant sections of the glossary for definitions of measures and methods of meta-analysis.

The discussion about the pros and cons of various accuracy measures is a never-ending story in which there is no consensus among experts and it is outside the remit of this book. To cut a long story short, sensitivity and specificity are often considered to be of a limited clinical value. For the question posed in this Case study, you are interested to discover the value of a negative endometrial ultrasound test (at a threshold of 5 mm thickness) for excluding endometrial cancer. This Case study describes the synthesis and interpretation using the likelihood ratio (LR) for a negative test result. For meta-analysis, it uses a bivariate model, an approach that provides robust summary accuracy estimates, although the description of its detail is outside the scope of this book.

Variation in test accuracy from study to study

The point estimate of accuracy in each study, its precision (confidence interval) and the possibility of heterogeneity can be explored by examining the variability of individual sensitivities and specificities in paired forest plots, which are provided in the published paper (not included in this Case study). Another graphical representation, specific to test accuracy meta-analyses, plots both sensitivity and specificity together in a single graph. The axes of this graph represent 1-specificity (x-axis) against sensitivity (y-axes). Known as the summary ROC (receiver operating characteristics) plot, it permits evaluation of the dispersion of individual study accuracy results. As shown in Box C4.7, there is a suspicion about heterogeneity because there is a wide dispersion of the accuracy results all over the space within the plot. When heterogeneity was found, its possible sources were searched for using subgroup

Sensitivity and **specificity**, measures of individual study accuracy, are often represented as paired forest plots to help appreciate the correlation between these indices. Increasing sensitivity values are frequently accompanied by decreasing specificities. This correlation makes it mandatory to meta-analyse both indices simultaneously in a bivariate model. If studies share the same positivity threshold, i.e. the cut-off to define a negative test result, the meta-analysis could calculate pooled sensitivity and specificity. Conversely, if studies used a variety of thresholds, calculating a pooled sensitivity and specificity does not make sense; a **summary ROC** (receiver operating characteristics) curve should be estimated instead.

Box C4.7 Exploring variation in individual accuracy results and summarizing them among studies evaluating endometrial ultrasound

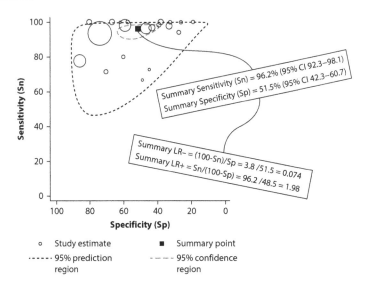

Summary Sensitivity (Sn) = 96.2% (95% CI 92.3–98.1)
Summary Specificity (Sp) = 51.5% (95% CI 42.3–60.7)

Summary LR– = (100-Sn)/Sp = 3.8 /51.5 = 0.074
Summary LR+ = Sn/(100-Sp) = 96.2 /48.5 = 1.98

○ Study estimate   ■ Summary point
····· 95% prediction   ─ ─ ─ 95% confidence
        region   region

Plot of sensitivity *versus* specificity

Sensitivities and specificities among studies with an endometrial ultrasound test threshold of 5 mm thickness are shown with empty circles. The summary estimate of sensitivity (96%; 95% confidence interval or CI 92–98%) and specificity (52%; 95% CI 42–61%) obtained using a bivariate model is shown with a filled square and its confidence area shown with a slashed ellipse around the square. Dotted ellipse shows the 95% prediction region that is interpreted as the region where the results of new studies could lie if they feature the same participants, index test and reference standard.

Based on Gynecol Oncol 2020; **157**: 624–633, doi: 10.1159/000520878.

analysis within the published paper (not reported here in detail) examining the impact of exclusion criteria based on the mean age of study participants, hormone replacement therapy or tamoxifen use, geographic region and publication date. No explanation for heterogeneity could be found in this paper.

Summary receiver operating characteristics curve (SROC) is a meta-analytic method of summarizing the performance of a dichotomous test, pooling 2×2 tables from multiple studies with different cut-off points. It takes into account the relation between test sensitivity and specificity among the individual studies by plotting the true positive rate (sensitivity) against the false positive rate (100-specificity).

Heterogeneity is the variation of accuracy between studies. It may arise because of differences between studies in key characteristics of their participants, index tests and reference standards (clinical heterogeneity), and their study designs and quality (methodological heterogeneity). Index test threshold variation is a key source of heterogeneity in test accuracy reviews.

Quantitative synthesis of results

In this instance, heterogeneity remains unexplained despite an exhaustive exploration. Now do we, or do we not, perform a meta-analysis? As discussed in Step 4, caution is required. In this review, the authors chose to pool sensitivities and specificities of individual studies using the same 5 mm thickness threshold. They use a bivariate random effects model which takes into account the correlation of both accuracy indices. Box C4.7 shows the accuracy of the 20 studies evaluating the accuracy of endometrial ultrasound at a 5 mm thickness threshold, deploying sensitivity and specificity. A meta-analysis using the bivariate model produced summary sensitivity and specificity from which LRs were derived: LR– was 0.074 (interestingly the summary LR+ for a positive test is 1.98 although this information was not really required to help with decision-making in your case scenario).

Bivariate model estimates the correlation between sensitivity and specificity and incorporates this in the meta-analysis of results from individual test accuracy studies.

Step 5: Interpreting the findings

The prevalence of endometrial cancer varies according to age. So, the likelihood or probability of cancer given a negative ultrasound test result will also vary. The changes in probability produced by the summary LR– can be mathematically computed or they can be estimated using a nomogram (see Box C4.8). A negative test result virtually eliminates

Box C4.8 The impact of a negative test result in endometrial ultrasound (at a 5 mm threshold) on the likelihood of endometrial cancer among postmenopausal women with vaginal bleeding

Generating post-test probabilities

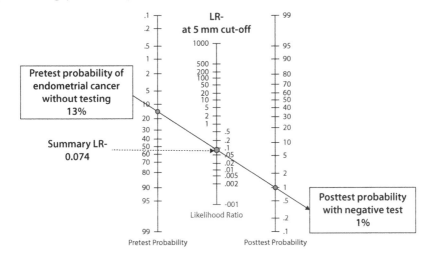

*Nomogram from N Engl J Med 1975; **293**: 257, doi: 10.1056/NEJM197507312930513.*

Post-test probabilities of endometrial cancer according to risk groups based on age

Age group	Pre-test probability*	Post-test probability+
<50 years	0.5%	0.04%
51–60 years	1.0%	0.08%
>60 years	13.0%	1.1%

Obtained from population-based data.

See Box C4.7 for the summary likelihood ratio for a negative test result, LR–.

+ *Computed using the following formula:*

$$Post\text{-}test\,probability = \frac{Likelihood\,ratio \times Pre\text{-}test\,probability}{[(1 - Pre\text{-}test\,probability) + (1 - Likelihood\,ratio)]}$$

the possibility of endometrial cancer among younger women; however, it may not substantially reduce the probability among older women (in our view).

Resolution of scenario

The answer to your question 'does a pelvic ultrasound scan exclude uterine cancer accurately in postmenopausal women with abnormal vaginal bleeding?' has to be 'yes, for many of your patients'. A negative result at less than 5 mm endometrial thickness rules out endometrial cancer with good certainty among low-risk patients (e.g. age < 60 years), so there should be no need for you to refer them to tertiary care. It is important to remember that there is always a chance of a false-negative test result, even among low-risk patients. So, if patients remain symptomatic, they will need further evaluation. For high-risk patients (e.g. age > 60 years), you don't have good certainty in ruling out disease from a negative ultrasound test, so you might even refer them to tertiary care without ultrasound testing. Needless to say, your low-risk patients with ultrasound endometrial thickness greater than 5 mm would need to be investigated further to ascertain the presence or absence of pathology in a tertiary care setting.

Pre-test probability is an estimate of the probability of disease before tests are carried out. It is usually based on disease prevalence.

Post-test probability is an estimate of the probability of disease in light of information obtained from testing. With accurate tests, the post-test estimates of probabilities change substantially from pre-test estimates.

Case study 5:
Reviewing qualitative evidence to evaluate patient experience

Step 1 Framing questions
↓
Step 2 Identifying relevant literature
↓
Step 3 Assessing the quality of the literature
↓
Step 4 Summarizing the evidence
↓
Step 5 Interpreting the findings

Elaine Denny

The purpose of qualitative research is to explore experience and to seek understanding and explanation. Through quantitative research, one may discover that an intervention is effective, but will patients find it acceptable? Will carers provide it? What will facilitate its implementation? What will hinder it? Answers to these and other related questions lie in the exploration of subjective experiences of people. There has been an increasing recognition within health that many issues such as the acceptability of interventions cannot fully be captured by quantitative means. Clinicians and practitioners need to allow people to relate their experiences and the way in which they interpret their world in order to understand their concerns better. Researchers need to study these subjective phenomena to help improve the insight practitioners and policymakers have. Thus there has been an increasing amount of health-related qualitative research and an interest in summarizing findings of qualitative papers in a rigorous way using the tools of systematic review, aiding evidence-based practice.

Primary qualitative research deals with very individual responses of study participants. This approach does not generate statistical averages and it can sometimes be erroneously assumed that this leads to problems in conducting systematic reviews. The reality is not so bleak. Systematic reviews can be used to integrate research findings in a structured way regardless of whether the primary studies are quantitative or qualitative. The results generated by individual qualitative studies can be collated and synthesized to gain new insights. Qualitative reviewers do this through metasynthesis, a technique that seeks to gain further understanding and explanations of the phenomena researched in primary studies.

This Case study will demonstrate how to employ reviews of qualitative research to enrich evidence-based medicine. It was developed as a learning aid in 2010 and remains pertinent for teaching and learning in the third edition of this book. We decided to retain this Case study in a form close to how it was presented in the second edition. It will demonstrate how the key points about appraisal shown at the end of each Step in this book can be employed to evaluate such reviews for their trustworthiness and usefulness.

Qualitative research seeks to understand the way people make sense of events and experiences.

Quantitative research involves the collection of data in numerical form, or that which can be converted to numeric form for analysis.

Metasynthesis: The synthesis of existing qualitative research findings on a specific research question. This does not involve meta-analysis.

DOI: 10.1201/9781003220039-12

Scenario: The experience of endometriosis

You are a general practitioner in a busy practice, and you have just had a long consultation with a young woman. She presented with chronic pelvic pain and also found sexual intercourse very painful, which was affecting her relationship with her partner. She told you that the pain was constantly there, although it was worse around menstruation, and that she was at the end of her tether. You knew from her records that over the years she had consulted with some of your colleagues who had prescribed non-steroidal anti-inflammatory analgesia and oral contraception, but nothing so far had relieved the pain. Your colleagues had suspected that she was exaggerating the pain associated with normal menstruation. When you questioned how long this had been going on, she replied that it had been 10 years. Having browsed the Internet, she suspected that her symptoms may be caused by endometriosis. You referred her to a gynaecologist, who carried out a laparoscopy. This confirmed the diagnosis of endometriosis. You wondered whether a referral could have been made earlier and if the delay in diagnosing endometriosis would affect her experience.

In order to feel better equipped to manage similar patients in the future, you decided to find out whether this woman's experience was typical of endometriosis. Qualitative research findings will elaborate on the experience of women with endometriosis. You search PubMed from the sources of reviews shown in Box 0.1. Typing the words 'endometriosis' AND 'qualitative research' in the query box and clicking the search button, there are 106 hits. You imagine that this large number of studies must have been summarized in a review, so you apply the systematic review filter in the above PubMed search. You find 22 citations. Reading through all titles and abstracts, you find that only two closely match your original query:

- Systematic reviews of qualitative evidence: What are the experiences of women with endometriosis? *J Obstet Gynaecol* 2006: **26**: 501–6, doi: 10.1080/01443610600797301.
- Women's experiences of endometriosis: A systematic review and synthesis of qualitative research. *J Fam Plann Reprod Health Care* 2015; **41**: 225–34, doi: 10.1136/jfprhc-2013-100853.

You decide to appraise the original review in detail first and then add the findings of the last review in the interpretation stage (Step 5).

Step 1: Framing the question

Free-form question

How does the experience of endometriosis impact on women's lives?

Question components

The participants: A clinically suitable sample of patients.

The interventions: Comparison of groups with and without the intervention.

The outcomes: Changes in health status, social relationships, self-image, etc. due to interventions.

The study design: Ways of conducting research.

Structured question

The participants   Women with a confirmed diagnosis of endometriosis.
The interventions   Either observation or treatment for endometriosis.
The outcomes   Effects on pain, work and social relationships,
                        self-image, etc.
The study design   Interviews, focus groups, diary keeping.

Note that the question does not pose a statistically testable hypothesis as the *outcomes* are described subjectively by study participants rather than quantified numerically.

Step 2: Identifying relevant studies

A search of PubMed using the search term endometriosis revealed 12,546 citations. The majority were reports of quantitative studies. Using filters for qualitative research to narrow the search to qualitative studies produced 192 citations. However, the majority of these papers did not have a qualitative methodology and endometriosis was not the primary focus of the research. From this search, only four papers fulfilled the selection criteria based on the structured question above. The major social science search engines were searched using the following key terms: endometriosis, pain, self-image and terms for qualitative methodology (Box C5.1). From these searches and reference lists, further four qualitative studies on living with endometriosis emerged, giving eight peer-reviewed studies for this review (Box C5.2).

As in all good reviews, the process concerning study selection and the decisions regarding selection should be transparent. In reviews of qualitative research, this is particularly important when different study

Identifying relevant literature
- Develop search term combinations
- Search relevant electronic databases
- Search other relevant resources
- Obtain full papers of potentially relevant citations
- Include/exclude studies using preset selection criteria

Study design filter employs a search term combination to capture citations of studies with a particular design.

Box C5.1 Some important databases and platforms for qualitative research in healthcare

ASSIA/PROQUEST

Applied Social Sciences Index and Abstracts is an indexing and abstracting database that covers health, social services, psychology, sociology, economics and politics.

PsycInfo

This is a database produced by the American Psychological Association and contains abstracts from all aspects of psychology.

EBSCO

This is a platform for full-text databases for psychology and the behavioural sciences.

Google Scholar

This broad, accessible and easy-to-use platform covers a range of disciplines and is useful for qualitative research.

Social Science Citation Index

This is accessed via the Web of Science and provides citation information that enables researchers to source research data.

Searching for qualitative studies

See Section 2.1.3 for searching for study designs. A qualitative research design filter can be used to restrict the citations of initial searches to those with a qualitative methodology. Owing to its in-depth thesaurus terms, CINAHL is generally accepted as a good database to find qualitative research articles. In CINAHL, exploding 'qualitative research' will include 'action research', 'ethnographic research', 'grounded theory', 'naturalistic inquiry' and 'phenomenological research'. Other terms that can be part of a qualitative research filter include: interviews.exp (includes a structured interview, semi-structured interview, unstructured interview); observational methods.exp (includes non-participant observation, participant observation); focus groups; narratives; and diary keeping.

Box C5.2 Identification of relevant literature on experiences of women with endometriosis

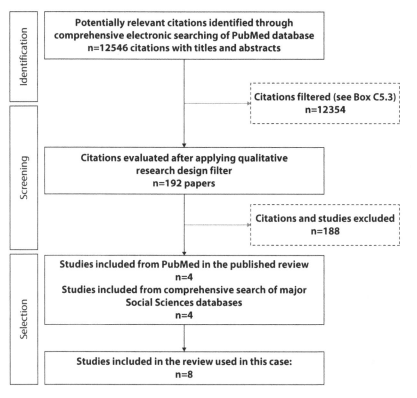

Based on J Obstet Gynaecol 2006: **26**: 501–6, doi: 10.1080/01443610600797301.

Box C5.3 Some important study designs for qualitative research in healthcare

Interviewing	Questioning people about their views or experience of a phenomenon or event. Can range from structured, where each participant is asked the same questions, to unstructured, which consists of a list of broad areas to be covered, the exact format of each interview being determined as it progresses.
Focus group	The collection of qualitative data using a group interview on a topic chosen by the researcher. Usually 6–12 people are involved, and they can be used to gauge issues of importance to interested parties in order to develop an interview schedule, or as a research method in their own right.
Diary keeping	A qualitative research method, usually an addition to questionnaire or interview data, where participants record experiences and emotions contemporaneously. Can be free form, where people write what they want to, or structured where they have specific questions to answer or topics to write about.

---

designs are to be considered simultaneously (Box C5.3). There is a debate around whether studies using different methods should be combined in a review, although some argue that such restrictions detract from the richness of data obtained. In this review, the selection was not restricted by the qualitative research method.

Step 3: Assessing study quality

There have been a number of methods developed to assess the quality of qualitative studies, although it is not appropriate to have a formulaic approach to determine the quality of this type of research.

In this review, the framework for the study of the quality assessment paid particular attention to the validity with which studies captured the meaning that women put on their experience. From this, an insight or understanding develops of the experience of endometriosis. A set of questions was formulated to be addressed when reading each of the articles in order to assess quality (Box C5.4). These need to be used with

The **quality** of a qualitative research study depends on the degree to which its design, conduct and analysis are trustworthy. Trustworthiness consists of several concepts including credibility, dependability, transferability, and confirmability.

Box C5.4 Description of quality of studies on experiences of women with endometriosis

Key issues on which the quality of qualitative research studies is judged

- Qualitative research gives a voice to participants, which allows them to talk about their experiences; therefore, research findings should reflect their perspective and not that of the researcher.
- Qualitative research design should be flexible enough for adaptation as perspectives of participants are revealed, but without losing rigour.

- The sample should be purposive, that is, drawn from the population that has the experience. However, it should not be so narrowly drawn that only certain experiences get reported. For example, sampling purely from self-help groups will often attract participants with negative experiences.
- Transparency in each stage of the research process is vital in a flexible and responsive research design.
- Various sources of knowledge are usually consulted for the literature review, and the extent to which the study under review conforms to or refutes this can be gauged.
- How the research moves through these stages should be explicit and justified. Often this will be an iterative process, in which case an explanation as to how each stage is influenced by the previous one should be given.
- Qualitative research is context specific and so the aim is to increase understanding. There should be a discussion of the extent to which the findings are consistent with those from similar studies.

Description of study quality

Information on quality is presented as 100% stacked bars. Data in the stacks represent the number of studies.

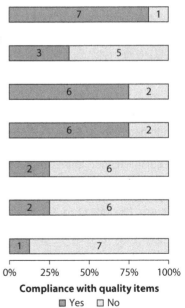

Based on J Obstet Gynaecol 2006; **26**: 501–6.

A guideline on Standards for Reporting Qualitative Research (SRQR) provides quality items for the assessment of qualitative studies (Acad Med 2014; **89**: 1245–51, doi: 10.1097/ACM.0000000000000388).

sensitivity in order to allow a qualitative critical appraisal. As this is a subjective process, it is crucial that quality assessment is initially undertaken by at least two reviewers acting independently, who then come together to formulate an agreed assessment. One important element of a systematic review of qualitative research is the notion of generalization (Box C5.4). Within qualitative research, the aim is not to extrapolate to wider populations, but to add to the understanding of a phenomenon. So in this case we would want to know how far the findings of the studies in the review concur with other studies that provide insight into the experience of endometriosis.

Step 4: Summarizing the evidence

The reporting of the narrative is a common method of presentation of findings in primary qualitative studies. In a systematic review, these can be collated and synthesized. This is usually accomplished by the generation of themes, which can initially be done by using the key areas identified within each selected study which is carried out by reviewing published findings, rather than re-analysing original data. Reading and re-reading the studies will result in the development and possible merging of further themes. This process can be facilitated by the use of qualitative data handling software (Box C5.5).

The themes formulated in this way allow the synthesis of the qualitative findings. This integration of studies is analogous to the pooling of data in a quantitative review. It is important that during this process the original meaning of the work is not lost. Similarities in the studies can

---

Box C5.5 A simple overview of qualitative data synthesis

- Data collected in qualitative research can include transcripts of interviews, group discussions, observation, photographs, reflective field notes, etc.
- The analysis of qualitative data involves the interpretation of these transcripts to form impressions. Coding is an interpretive technique that requires the researcher to read the text and demarcate segments within it. Each segment is labelled with a word or short phrase that suggests how the associated data segments inform the research objectives. To ensure rigour, this process is often carried out separately by two or more researchers. When coding is complete, the researcher can discuss similarities and differences in codes across transcripts. This forms the basis for organizing and reporting results.
- The use of qualitative data handling software can assist in the analysis of large quantities of data, by categorizing it according to codes generated by the researcher. This way data on a particular phenomenon can be retrieved quickly from every transcript.
- Using the example of endometriosis pain, all references to pain in the interview transcripts may be entered into the software under the code of 'pain'. Sub codes of 'pelvic pain', 'dyspareunia', etc. may also be used to categorize the data. The researcher can later retrieve all references to pain from the entire participant group at the click of a mouse.

be identified and categorized using the identified or emergent themes. Aberrant findings, that is, those findings which are not consistent with the identified themes, can be explored to elicit an explanation. In this way, a reviewer gets a picture of the phenomenon under study, in this case the experience of living with endometriosis.

The reliability of summarizing qualitative evidence and interpretation of findings (Steps 4 and 5) can be improved in one of two ways. Where there is a research team, each member conducts Steps 4 and 5 independently. They will then agree on emerging themes and iron out inconsistencies, which need to be made transparent in subsequent reports or publications. Alternatively, Steps 4 and 5 can be independently verified by someone outside of the team who has expertise in the research issue.

In the endometriosis studies reviewed, a detailed narrative was reported but analysis of the data was limited. Common themes were identified from the articles, but no article reported on all of these themes apart from pain. Nevertheless, similar results were reported by all studies. As pain was the one common theme, it provides a useful example of how findings can be synthesized. Various descriptions of pain were given in the articles. In three of these articles, individual narrative from participants in the research was reported in the words of the author(s) as representative of the group as a whole. The remaining papers gave examples of descriptions of pain from individual women, with terms such as 'intense', 'a knife going into each ovary', 'stabbing' and 'tremendous' frequently used. This is unlikely to be captured by the linear pain scales of quantitative research.

In synthesizing this information, we can conclude that pain was a constant theme in all qualitative research on endometriosis. In three studies, this was described by the authors from unreported data, but five studies reported women's own descriptions of the quality and severity of pain. Seven of the studies also reported how the experience of pain impacted on the quality of life, e.g. on work and social relationships. In four of the studies, women described how their social life had suffered, with friends and family losing patience when planned events were continually cancelled. Relationships with partners were also negatively affected, although one study did point to partners as offering the major support to women with endometriosis. Three studies found that women who took time off work due to pain felt guilty and were often disbelieved by colleagues and employers, sometimes being made to feel they were malingering.

Phenomenon is an occurrence or a fact. It is often used as a generic term for the object of a research study.

Theme is an idea that is developed by the coding of qualitative data. The large quantities of data produced by a qualitative study are managed by the generation of themes and the coding of parts of the data to each theme. The perspectives of each research participant on each theme can be compared and analysed.

Step 5: Interpreting the findings

This Case scenario focused on the experience of endometriosis reported in a systematic review of qualitative research. It revealed that the experience of endometriosis has a profound negative effect on the lives of women. Despite a comprehensive search of relevant databases, only a few studies of variable quality were found. They provided a detailed narrative but analyses were limited. As one purpose of qualitative research is the generation of a new theory to explain a phenomenon, this lack of analysis is a limitation of the reviewed research.

Adding the findings from the other review your own search had captured (*J Fam Plann Reprod Health Care* 2015; **41**: 225–34), you recognize that the key themes are about improving your own education about a comprehensive approach to pain and endometriosis. Evidence gaps were also identified in the areas of experiences of endometriosis-associated infertility and the impact of reduced social participation.

Theory is abstract knowledge or reasoning as a way of explaining social relations. Theory may influence research (deduction), or research may lead to the development of the theory (induction).

Resolution of scenario

By appraising the systematic reviews, you have gained a better understanding of your own patient's lived experience, located within the broader context of endometriosis experience, and have discovered that her history is a familiar one. You could not have gained this insight by reading clinical papers that focus on the effectiveness of different treatments rather than on the impact of living with endometriosis. Your understanding of women's experiences has improved and this may influence your management of similar patients in the future.

Case study 6:
Reviewing the effects of educational interventions

••

Sharon Buckley

Health professions educators use systematic reviews to evaluate the effects of educational interventions. Peculiarities of electronic databases and the inherent complexity of primary educational research make systematic reviews in this field challenging. However, such reviews can provide valuable insights into the available evidence about particular effects of teaching methods on student learning, guiding resource allocation and supporting educational practice.

This Case study will explore the specific issues relating to systematic reviews of the effects of educational interventions. Based on a published review, it will consider requirements for literature searching and quality assessment in the educational context. It was developed as a learning aid in 2010 and remains pertinent for teaching and learning in the third edition of this book. We decided to retain this Case study in a form close to how it was presented in the second edition. It will demonstrate an approach to the synthesis of educational research evidence when meta-analysis is not appropriate.

Scenario: Effects of portfolios on student learning in undergraduate medical education

You are an Education Development Specialist based in a large medical and nursing school. Your faculty is considering introducing a professional development portfolio for all its undergraduate medical students. Views on whether, how and when the portfolio should be introduced are mixed: some faculty view portfolios as ideal preparation for postgraduate medical education and lifelong learning, while others as a drain on scarce resources that emphasizes reflection at the expense of essential clinical knowledge and understanding.

You are keen that any decisions about curriculum development should be based on the best available evidence as to the effects of using a portfolio on undergraduate student learning. You search PubMed from the sources of reviews shown in Box 0.1. Typing the words 'student portfolio' in the query box and clicking the search button, there are 799 hits. You imagine that this large number of studies must have been summarized in a review, so you apply the Systematic review filter in the above PubMed search. You find nine citations. Reading through all titles and abstracts,

| Step 1 |
| Framing questions |
| ↓ |
| Step 2 |
| Identifying relevant literature |
| ↓ |
| Step 3 |
| Assessing the quality of the literature |
| ↓ |
| Step 4 |
| Summarizing the evidence |
| ↓ |
| Step 5 |
| Interpreting the findings |

Best Evidence Medical and Health Professions Education (BEME): An international collaboration committed to the development of evidence-informed education in the health professions through the production and dissemination of educational reviews. BEME also aims to foster a culture of best evidence medical education amongst individuals, institutions and national bodies (bemecollaboration. org).

DOI: 10.1201/9781003220039-13

you identify the following Best Evidence Medical Education (BEME) review that is relevant to your search:

- The educational effects of portfolios on undergraduate student learning: A Best Evidence Medical Education (BEME) systematic review. *Med Teacher* 2009; **31**: 282–98, doi: 10.1080/01421590902889897.

You appraise the review so that you can be confident in using its conclusions to inform your practice.

Step 1: Framing the question

Free-form question

How does the use of portfolios affect student learning in undergraduate health professions education?

Structured question

		Question components
Participants	Undergraduates, defined as students following a course of initial training in a particular profession leading to a degree qualification.	**The participants:** A suitable sample of learners.
Intervention	A 'portfolio', defined as a collection of evidence of student learning, a learning journal or diary, or a combination of these two elements.	**The intervention:** An educational intervention.
Outcomes	Educational outcomes can be grouped according to the nature of learning. In the Kirkpatrick evaluation model as adapted for use in health professions education, educational outcomes are grouped into: learner reactions to participation or completion of the educational intervention, modification of learner attitudes or perceptions, modification of knowledge or skills, change in learner behaviour and change in delivery of care and health outcomes. This review collected information on any reported outcome demonstrating an effect on student learning as a result of using a portfolio. Changes in delivery of care or improvements in patient outcomes are not normally demonstrable outcomes for undergraduate education as students are not responsible for the provision of patient care.	**The outcomes:** Change(s) in perceptions, attitudes, knowledge, skills, behaviour, etc. due to interventions. **The study design:** A way of conducting research to assess the effect of educational intervention(s) on outcomes.
Study designs	Primary research studies of all types that assess the learning outcomes following the use of a portfolio.	

The reviewers clearly defined their participants, interventions and outcomes but have not limited the review to studies looking at particular outcomes or study designs. They wished to ensure that relevant studies were not missed by prematurely excluding particular outcomes or study designs. Given the variety of educational research designs and the range of learning outcomes associated with port-folios reported anecdotally, you are satisfied that this approach is appropriate.

While the published review includes studies from professions allied to medicine such as dentistry and physiotherapy, this case study will focus solely on medicine and nursing, which have the largest body of available evidence.

Step 2: Identifying the literature

Searches of the educational literature for medicine and allied profes-sions can be challenging. The relevant educational literature is dispersed across many different databases, subject headings vary considerably and the classification of articles against subject headings is not always accurate. The use of subject headings only may not reliably find all rel-evant articles, and therefore free text words also were used. To ensure comprehensive coverage, reviewers searched 10 different databases from their inception and without language restriction, encompassing the literature from educational (ERIC, British and Australian Education Indices), clinical (Medline, Embase, Cinahl, BNI) and social sciences (ASSIA, PsycInfo) (Boxes 2.2, C5.1 and C6.1). Search terms and synonyms used reflect closely the participants and intervention components of the research question and the reviewers used both subject headings and free text (Box C6.2). The reviewers supplemented the electronic searches with hand searches of the reference lists of selected studies.

Box C6.1 Searching for medical education literature

Some important databases of medical education research (see also Boxes 2.2 and C5.1)

BNI (about.proquest.com/en/products-services/bni)

The British Nursing Index is a database for support of the practice, education and research for nurses, midwives and health providers.

ASSIA (about.proquest.com/en/products-services/ ASSIA-Applied-Social-Sciences-Index-and-Abstracts)

Applied Social Sciences Index and Abstracts is an indexing and abstracting database that covers health, social services, psychology, sociology, economics, politics, race relations and education.

ERIC (eric.ed.gov)

The Education Resources Information Centre is an online library of education research and information sponsored by the US Institute of Education Sciences.

BEI (ebsco.com/products/research-databases/british-education-index)

The British Education Index covers all aspects of educational policy and administration, evaluation and assessment, technology and special educational needs.

AEI (pq-static-content.proquest.com/collateral/media2/documents/australian_education_index.pdf)

The Australian Education Index is a subscription database produced by the Cunningham Library at the Australian Council for Education Research. It covers topics relating to trends and practices in teaching, learning and educational management.

TIMELIT (timelit.org)

Topics in Medical Education, a database covering professional education, health education and patient education.

Identification of relevant literature on educational effects of portfolios

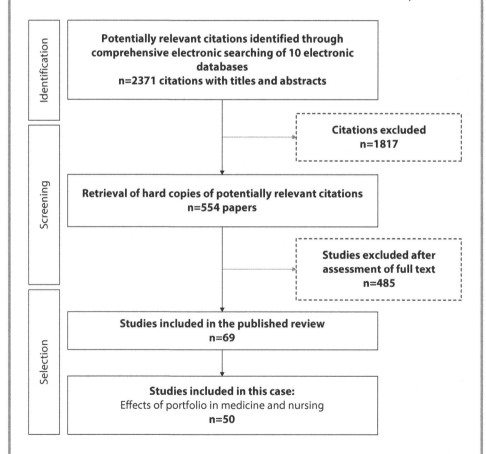

The BEME Collaboration has produced a range of guides on how to conduct an educational systematic review, including appropriate methods for searching the medical and health professions education literature, available at: bemecollaboration.org/Publications+Research+Methodology/

Box C6.2 How to develop a search term combination for searching electronic bibliographic databases

An example of a search term combination for Medline database

Free-form question: How does the use of portfolios affect student learning in undergraduate (medical and nursing) education?

Structured question (not all components may be needed for searching)

- The participants   Undergraduate medical and nursing education
- The intervention   Portfolio
- The outcome   Any (not used in search term combination)
- The study design   Any (not used in search term combination)

Question components and relevant search terms	Type of terms MeSH	Free	Boolean operator
The participants: Undergraduates			
1 students	x		
2 freshers		x	
3 freshman/men		x	
4 Sophomore		x	OR (captures *participants*)
5 Senior		x	
6 additional terms (see in original report of the review)			
7 OR 1-6			
The participants: Health education			
8 medical education, undergraduate	x		
9 clinical skills	x		
10 allied health	x		
11 nursing	x		
12 pharmacology	x		OR (captures *participants*)
13 medical		x	
14 clinical teaching		x	
15 additional terms (see in original report of the review)			
16 OR 8-15			
The intervention: Portfolio			
17 portfolio		x	
18 learning record		x	
19 case folder		x	
20 case notes		x	OR (captures *intervention*)
21 learning journal		x	

Question components and relevant search terms	Type of terms		Boolean operator
	MeSH	Free	
22 log book		x	
23 self reflection		x	
24 additional terms (see in original report of the review)			
25 OR 17-24			
26 **AND /7,16,25**			AND (combines all components above)

See related sections in Step 2.

The relevance of grey literature to educational systematic reviews depends very much on the topic being examined. For this review, the reviewers judged at an early stage that unpublished sources were unlikely to yield significant papers not found by other methods and that searching of the grey literature would be a poor use of time and resources. Whilst this approach may be appropriate in this case, other reviews may require a search of the grey literature.

Screening of the 2371 possible citations identified 580 as possibly relevant using predefined selection criteria based on the review question. Of these, full papers of 554 were obtained. Further screening of full manuscripts against the selection criteria identified 69 studies for inclusion, 18 from medicine, 32 from nursing and 19 from other professions (Box C6.1). Selection criteria were established *a priori* and applied by two independent reviewers. Reasons for exclusion were primarily that a particular intervention did not meet the definition of a portfolio or that the study did not contain primary research data.

Aware of the particular factors relating to educational literature, you agree that the reviewers' approach to searching and selection is appropriate and, as far as possible, avoids the risk of missing studies due to publication bias.

Step 3: Assessing study quality

Among the 18 studies in medicine, there were two with a comparative design, including one randomized trial, and 16 observational studies without a comparison group. Among the 32 nursing studies, there were also two with a comparative design but without randomization, and 29 observational studies without a comparison group. Whilst many studies used a combination of methods, over half of all included studies administered questionnaires to learners; a third used focus group interviews of learners, and another third performed direct assessment of portfolios. For educational studies, assessment of study quality is a controversial area, with conflicting views on the appropriateness of particular quality assessment tools. Here, the reviewers assembled a quality checklist and applied this to all studies, regardless of design. In many included studies, it was not possible

Triangulation is the application and combination of several research methodologies in the study of the same phenomenon.

Box C6.3 Description of quality of studies on educational effects of portfolios

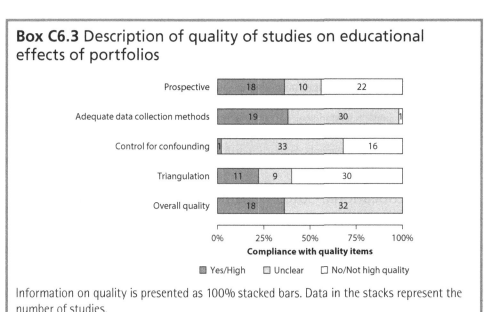

Information on quality is presented as 100% stacked bars. Data in the stacks represent the number of studies.

to make a judgement about study quality due to a lack of clarity in reporting. As an example, Box C6.3 illustrates data for four of the 11 quality items used. The reviewers called, as have other commentators on educational research, for authors to report their methods more thoroughly. However, the review also reported an encouraging trend: in each professional group (medicine and nursing), more recent studies had significantly higher quality scores than those published earlier (data not shown). Overall, 18 of the 50 studies included in the review were classed as higher quality, meeting seven or more of the 11 quality items. The higher quality group included one randomized controlled trial, in which medical students taking a clinical oncology module were randomly allocated to either receive a portfolio or to a control group without a portfolio. The portfolio group recorded patient encounters and received tutorial support in portfolio development.

Step 4: Summarizing the evidence

For this review, as for many other educational systematic reviews, the limitations of the available data meant that meta-analysis of data and statistical investigation of heterogeneity in effects between studies was inappropriate and that a descriptive approach to summarizing the evidence was needed. The reviewers adopted a twofold approach to this.

First, the reviewers described how portfolios are used in undergraduate education. Portfolios were mainly used in the clinical setting and their completion was compulsory for students. They required the students to reflect on their learning and share their reflections with other students and staff. In general, students had only a limited choice of content and were assessed on their work. Learning journals or diaries were common in nursing, with 'hybrid' portfolios that combined collections of evidence with a learning journal more common in medicine.

Second, the reviewers identified the main messages emerging from the 'higher quality' studies, providing the reader with a rich description of the findings of these studies, grouped according to the theme (Box C6.4). Higher quality studies reported that using a portfolio can enhance students' knowledge and understanding, particularly their ability to integrate theory with practice, but that these improvements do not always translate into improved assessments. Similarly, portfolios can encourage

---

Box C6.4 Educational outcomes among studies of portfolios

Key themes recorded in higher quality studies

Portfolios may:

- Improve students' knowledge and understanding, especially their ability to integrate theory with practice. However, these effects may not always translate into higher scores in formal assessments
- Encourage students' self-awareness and reflection. However, keeping a portfolio will not, in itself, guarantee the *quality* of those reflections
- Assist tutors in providing structured feedback to their students and increase their awareness of students' needs
- Provide emotional support for students facing difficult situations such as a patient death
- Prepare students for the demands of postgraduate training
- Detract from other clinical learning, if implemented in such a way that the time required for completion is disproportionate.

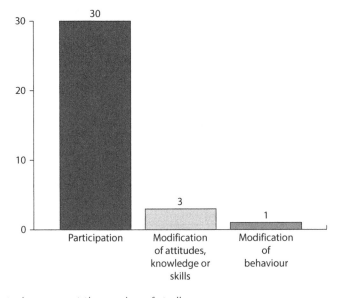

Data in the stacks represent the number of studies.

self-awareness and reflection but do not guarantee the quality of those reflections. Completing a portfolio can help some students to cope with difficult or uncertain situations, such as a patient death, and can prepare them for the rigours of postgraduate training. Engaging with students through a portfolio can help tutors become more aware of students' learning needs, influencing their teaching approaches and allowing them to give more structured feedback. Higher quality studies identified the time required for completion as the main drawback to portfolios. In some cases, where this detracts from other clinical learning, this is not desirable.

The effects of an educational intervention can be grouped using the Kirkpatrick model as modified for use in educational settings (Box C6.4). In this review, most studies demonstrated outcomes relating to participants' reactions to the portfolio or to changes in their knowledge, skills or attitudes. Only one study (from nursing) reported a change in participant behaviour.

Step 5: Interpreting the findings

This review showed that the available evidence for the educational effects of portfolios on student learning is limited. Relatively few studies were of higher methodological quality and most outcomes were related to learner reactions to participation in the intervention or change in knowledge, skills or attitudes, with only one study reporting a change in learner behaviour as a result of completing a portfolio. However, limited evidence is not synonymous with a lack of effectiveness. The summary of the evidence available does suggest that some important benefits in participants' perceptions, knowledge and skills are possible if portfolios are implemented appropriately. The reviewers made it clear that in order to realize the benefits of portfolios, the time demands on both students and tutors should be kept within reasonable limits. They also cautioned faculty against assuming that a portfolio will automatically develop students' reflective abilities and suggested that additional guidance on how to reflect should accompany any portfolio intervention that aims to develop these skills. Clearly, more research is needed, as is greater clarity and thoroughness of reporting, although the trend towards improvements in quality scores in more recent publications is encouraging.

Resolution of scenario

You are disappointed, but not surprised that the evidence base for the effectiveness of portfolios is limited, and are encouraged by the clear directions for implementation offered by the higher quality studies. You share the findings with faculty in your department and develop a proposal for implementation that incorporates the recommendations of the reviewers. You decide to include in your proposal a research study that measures directly the educational effects of portfolios, in order to add to the evidence base on the subject.

Case study 7: *To use or not to use a therapy? Incorporating evidence on harmful outcomes*

Katja Suter

Step 1
Framing questions
↓
Step 2
Identifying relevant literature
↓
Step 3
Assessing the quality of the literature
↓
Step 4
Summarizing the evidence
↓
Step 5
Interpreting the findings

Adverse effect is undesirable and unintended unpleasant or harmful *outcomes* resulting from an *intervention*.

For making informed decisions, healthcare professionals and patients need to balance the expected benefits against the potential harms of interventions. Thus, as well as covering beneficial outcomes, systematic reviews of effectiveness should include information on adverse effects and harms. But often the primary studies included in reviews do not capture data on the harmful outcomes at all, or they report this information sparingly. To allow the collation of information on rare harmful outcomes, particularly those that develop over a long time period, systematic reviews may include a range of study *designs* (as in Case study 2). Furthermore, systematic reviews may be developed exclusively to report on adverse effects.

This Case study demonstrates how to seek and assess evidence on harmful *outcomes* associated with drug therapies. Package leaflets of drugs or information for the user that accompany medicinal products often report long lists of potential adverse effects of varying frequency and severity. Reviews covering evidence on *all* possible adverse effects are not always necessary or feasible. Focusing on a *few* adverse effects, particularly those that are relevant for clinical decision-making, facilitates the comparison of expected benefits against potential harms. This Case study will evaluate potential harms associated with a drug treatment of known, well-established effectiveness. Based on a published review, it will apply the review theory related to framing questions, assessing study quality, summarizing the results on harmful effects and gauging the strength of the evidence on the treatment options, showing how to come up with a decision.

Scenario: Considering harmful outcomes when choosing an antihypertensive treatment

You currently have an overweight 50-year-old patient with recently diagnosed hypertension (150/100 mmHg) in your general practice. The blood pressure did not improve under the initial management strategy encouraging him to lose weight with lifestyle changes. You and your patient share the decision to start an antihypertensive treatment. Among the many drugs recommended in clinical practice guidelines, you prefer a renin-system blocking drug, either angiotensin-converting-enzyme

DOI: 10.1201/9781003220039-14

153

inhibitors (ACE-Is) or angiotensin-receptor blockers (ARBs). Which one to choose? The answer requires a comparison of relative benefits *versus* harms. Large trials have investigated the effects of ACE-Is and ARBs. You are aware that the two drugs are regarded as being equivalent in their effectiveness, e.g. their performance is similar in terms of *outcomes* such as major cardiovascular morbidity and mortality. You want to explore adverse effects, and you consult the following review:

● Updated report on comparative effectiveness of ACE inhibitors, ARBs, and direct renin inhibitors for patients with essential hypertension: much more data, little new information. *J Gen Intern Med* 2012; **27**: 716–29, doi: 10.1007/s11606-011-1938-8.

This review included experimental and observational studies directly comparing ACE-Is with ARBs, with a minimum study duration of 12 weeks and a comprehensive list of adverse effects was reported.

Step 1: Framing the question

Free-form question

Is there a difference in harms between ARBs and ACE-Is?

Structured question

The populations   Adults with essential hypertension.

The interventions   All drugs from the class of ARBs (e.g. losartan, irbesartan, valsartan or telmisartan) compared to drugs from the class of ACE-Is (e.g. captopril, enalapril, ramipril or fosinopril).

The outcomes   Cough and withdrawal due to adverse events.

The study designs   Experimental and observational studies with control groups (this Case study focuses on evidence collated from cohort and case-control studies).

> **Clinically relevant outcome** measurements directly measure how patients feel, what their function is or if they survive, focusing on what is critical and important.

Not all harmful *outcomes* have the same impact on decision-making. Ranking of beneficial and harmful *outcomes* according to their importance for the decision-making process facilitates the delineation of the structured question in a systematic review. Clinically relevant *outcomes* should be more important than surrogate measurements. In the classification proposed by the GRADE working group, all *outcomes* are classified into one of three categories according to their importance for decision-making: critical, important and not important. More common ones tend to play a more significant role in patient care than rare or very rare ones, even if the latter are more serious. Considering patient preferences, (very) rare effects are less likely to prevent us from recommending a drug of known, well-established effectiveness. According to a suggested scale, adverse effects can occur very frequently (more than 1 in 10); frequently (between 1 in 10 and 1 in 100);

> **Surrogate** outcome measurements substitute for direct measures of how patients feel, what their function is or if they survive. They include physiological variables or measures of subclinical disease. To be valid, the surrogate must be statistically correlated with the clinically relevant outcome.

occasionally (between 1 in 100 and 1 in 1000); rarely (between 1 in 1000 and 1 in 10,000); and very rarely (less than 1 in 10,000, including singular reports). Reversibility on discontinuation of medication is another feature of adverse effects. Obviously, frequent and non-reversible adverse effects will be critical, and infrequent and fully reversible adverse effects will not be important. Important adverse effects will sit somewhere between these two ends of the spectrum.

This Case study is restricted to two important harmful *outcomes*: cough and withdrawals due to adverse effects – these two outcomes are classified as important for decision-making. For simplicity, this Case study is also restricted to evaluating the potential harms with observational evidence. Since observational studies are often the only source of information on harmful *outcomes*, this Case study shows how to assess such evidence. Of course, in real life if experimental evidence is available, we would base our decisions on this because of its inherent lower risk of bias (Box 1.4).

Withdrawal of participants or patients can be for many reasons, e.g. non-compliance with the intervention, crossover to an alternative intervention, drop out of the study and loss to follow-up. When the reason for withdrawal is the appearance of an adverse effect, this information can be used as an *outcome* measure for drug safety.

Step 2: Identifying relevant literature

Capturing studies reporting on harmful *outcomes* of drug therapies is challenging as standardized reporting is not the norm. Reporting guidelines covering harms in randomized trials and systematic reviews have relatively recently been published (*BMJ* 2016; **352**: i157, doi:10.1136/bmj.i157), so it will take a while before they are applied across the board. Furthermore, the MeSH term 'Drug-Related Side Effects and Adverse Reactions' was introduced only in 2014.

The review used search terms for hypertension (*participants*), drug *interventions* and applicable study *designs* to search Medline, Embase, the Cochrane Central Register of Controlled Trials, the register of the Cochrane Hypertension Review Group and grey literature sources (e.g. regulatory data, clinical trial registries and conference abstracts). The search provided 2090 citations, the screening of titles/abstracts narrowed the results down to 328 citations for full-text assessments, and the final study pool for the systematic review included 110 reports (Box C7.1). Of those, 39 experimental and three observational studies reported on cough and 39 experimental and two observational studies on withdrawals due to adverse effects.

Step 3: Assessing study quality

Study design threshold for study selection

Different study *designs* need to be considered for information about harmful *outcomes* as this evidence from randomized trials is often missing. Randomized trials are well suited for common, anticipated adverse

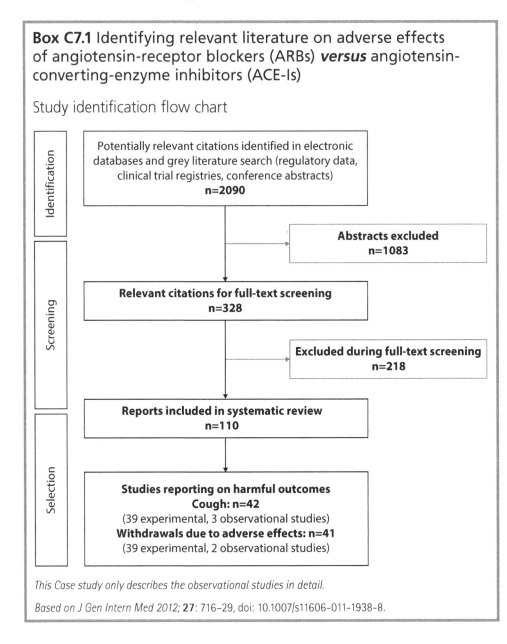

Box C7.1 Identifying relevant literature on adverse effects of angiotensin-receptor blockers (ARBs) *versus* angiotensin-converting-enzyme inhibitors (ACE-Is)

Study identification flow chart

Identification

Potentially relevant citations identified in electronic databases and grey literature search (regulatory data, clinical trial registries, conference abstracts)
n=2090

Abstracts excluded
n=1083

Screening

**Relevant citations for full-text screening
n=328**

**Excluded during full-text screening
n=218**

**Reports included in systematic review
n=110**

Selection

**Studies reporting on harmful outcomes
Cough: n=42**
(39 experimental, 3 observational studies)
Withdrawals due to adverse effects: n=41
(39 experimental, 2 observational studies)

This Case study only describes the observational studies in detail.

Based on J Gen Intern Med 2012; 27: 716–29, doi: 10.1007/s11606-011-1938-8.

effects, whereas observational studies may be more useful for delayed or rare adverse effects. It is advisable to include different observational study *designs*, taking into account the strengths and weaknesses of each (Box 1.4). The review underlying this Case study included randomized trials and observational (cohort and case-control) studies. This Case study only explores the assessment of observational data.

Quality assessment of observational studies on harmful outcomes

Quality assessment of observational studies is concerned with methodological issues important for establishing comparable groups to prevent selection bias, ensuring the capture of information concerning the use of (or, in other words, *exposure* to) the *interventions*, minimizing bias in the measurement of *outcomes*, and an appropriate statistical analysis. The key quality items used in this case study are described below.

Prospective design: A prospective design with forward planning, comprehensive assessment of the patients and collection of all relevant data may facilitate efforts outlined above to minimize bias (Box C2.2). One might have access to a database which has already meticulously documented the enrolment of patients, carefully measured a wide variety of prognostic factors, and followed up all patients and rigorously recorded their outcomes. In this situation, a retrospective design will not be a particular disadvantage. A prospective study, badly done, may fail to document how patients were selected, measure prognostic factors in an incomplete and sloppy way, and lose a large proportion of their patients to follow-up. Therefore, prospective or retrospective should not be treated as quality criteria in themselves. In addition, one should look to see whether studies adhered to the criteria listed above.

Assembling comparable groups at the outset: Groups that are unequal in important prognostic factors pose a major threat to the validity of observational studies. This is because those differences – rather than the differences in the interventions – may be linked to the outcomes. (Large) randomized studies balance out potential confounding factors by randomly allocating patients with varying risk factors equally between groups. Assembling groups that are similar at baseline is more challenging in observational studies, and in most cases analytical strategies with statistical adjustment for group differences are applied. To do so, the researchers have to identify at baseline all relevant prognostic factors and co-morbidities that can bring about harmful effects regardless of the *exposure*; avoiding ACE-Is in patients with chronic bronchitis as cough may be an adverse effect of ACE-I. This selective prescribing behaviour could bias the assessment of the frequency of cough.

Ascertaining exposure: In observational studies, it is essential to correctly identify those exposed and those not exposed to an intervention. Consider a study that included new and current users of antihypertensive drugs. More 'new users' of antihypertensive drugs were in the ACE-I group, while more 'previous users' of antihypertensive drugs entered the ARB group. A considerable proportion of those 'previous users' had experienced cough using ACE-Is and had switched to ARBs before entering the study. This could reduce the frequency of cough associated with ACE-Is. Thus it is important to minimize misclassification in *exposure*, by collecting information on all co-medications and any cross-over of medications.

The **quality** of a study depends on the degree to which its design, conduct and analysis minimize **biases**.

Bias leads to either overestimating or underestimating the 'true' impact of an intervention.

Confounding is a situation in comparative studies where the effect of an *exposure* or *intervention* on an *outcome* is distorted due to the association of the *outcome* with another factor, which can prevent or cause the *outcome* independent of the *exposure* or *intervention*. Data analysis may be adjusted for confounding in observational studies for known and measured confounding factors.

Outcome ascertainment: *Outcome* assessment in observational studies is vulnerable to the same biases as in experimental studies. Measurement bias has to be dealt with using similar precautions. Subjective outcomes such as a bothersome cough or the experience of other adverse effects that warranted withdrawal demand the person ascertaining the outcome be kept blind to the *exposure* status. Only a few observational studies manage to implement appropriate measures to achieve blinding. Adverse effects with less frequent or delayed occurrence need a (sufficiently) long follow-up for detection.

Appropriate analysis: Once key relevant prognostic factors have been identified, an appropriate adjustment in the analysis for differences of those factors between the groups increases the chance that any observed association between *exposure* and *outcome* reflects the 'truth'. It is often difficult to identify and adjust for *all* confounding factors. Loss to follow-up and missing values interfere with performing appropriate analysis.

> **Prognosis** is a probable course or outcome of a disease. **Prognostic factors** are patient or disease characteristics that influence the course. A good prognosis is associated with a low rate of undesirable outcomes. A poor prognosis is associated with a high rate of undesirable outcomes.

Description of quality of the included observational studies

A separate description of quality assessment of the two outcomes cough and withdrawal due to adverse effects is provided (Box C7.2). The quality of the assessment of different outcomes may differ, even if they are measured in the same studies. While cough is a subjective outcome susceptible to bias in the absence of blinding, the outcome withdrawal is objective and the absence of blinding is unlikely to influence the count of people who withdraw. Lack of blinded *outcome* assessment would be a limitation of the study quality for cough but it would not be for counting the number of withdrawals due to adverse effects.

The three cohort studies reporting on cough had considerable methodological weaknesses: Owing to the observational design, all studies were open label; patients, healthcare providers and outcome assessors were aware of the treatment allocations except in one study where the telephone interviewer who did the outcome assessment was blinded. All studies lacked conclusive information about co-morbidities and co-medication. Most studies did not report on loss to follow-up. Overall, the quality of the three observational studies was rated as poor.

Two observational studies (one cohort study and one case-control study) reporting on withdrawals due to adverse effects, too, had profound weaknesses. While some quality issues, e.g. blinding, were difficult or impossible to address, others would have been amenable to methodological safeguards, such as the case-control study could have described its selection of cases and controls. Both studies lacked information about patient characteristics, co-morbidities, co-medication and adjustment for differences in prognostic factors. Furthermore, they reported that significant amounts of data were missing and there was a considerable loss to follow-up. Overall, the quality of the three observational studies was rated as poor.

Box C7.2 Description of quality of comparative observational studies on adverse effects of angiotensin-receptor blockers (ARBs) versus angiotensin-converting-enzyme inhibitors (ACE-Is) in essential hypertension

Cough

Withdrawals for adverse effects

Compliance with quality items

■ Yes   □ Unclearly reported   □ No

This Case study only describes the observational studies. Data in stacks represent the number of studies.

Based on J Gen Intern Med 2012; 27: 716–29, doi: 10.1007/s11606-011-1938-8 and the previous review by the Agency for Healthcare Research and Quality (AHRQ) available at effectivehealthcare. ahrq.gov/products/ace-inhibitor-arb-2007/research-2007-1

Newcastle-Ottawa Scale (NOS) is a generic checklist for quality assessment of observational studies (ohri.ca/Programs/clinical_epidemiology/oxford.asp).

Step 4: Summarizing the evidence

Cough

Three cohort studies reported on cough: one large post-marketing cohort study with more than 50,000 patients and two smaller studies with 449 and 49 patients, respectively. Among a total of 51,908 patients, there were 691 cough events. The pooled summary estimate for ARBs to reduce cough compared to ACE-Is was an odds ratio (OR) of 0.40 with a 95% confidence interval of 0.34–0.48, without heterogeneity (I² 0%) (Box C7.3).

> **Odds ratio (OR)** is an effect measure for binary data. It is the ratio of odds in the experimental group to the odds in the control group.

Withdrawal due to adverse effects

One cohort and one case-control study reported on withdrawals due to adverse effects. Both studies were small with 39 and 88 patients, respectively. The two studies with this outcome found 18 withdrawals in 127 patients. After pooling, the point estimate described a large effect and an OR of 0.36, but the 95% confidence interval ranged from

---

Box C7.3 Forest plot for outcomes cough and withdrawal due to adverse effects comparing angiotensin-receptor blockers (ARBs) *versus* angiotensin-converting-enzyme inhibitors (ACE-Is)

Outcome: Cough

Study or Subgroup	ARB Events	Total	ACE-I Events	Total	Weight	Peto Odds Ratio Fixed, 95% CI
Gregoire 2001	4	80	55	369	5.6%	0.42 [0.21, 0.86]
Mackay 1999	64	14522	566	36888	94.0%	0.41 [0.34, 0.48]
Sato 2003	0	26	2	23	0.4%	0.11 [0.01, 1.88]
Total (95% CI)		**14628**		**37280**	**100.0%**	**0.40 [0.34, 0.48]**
Total events	68		623			

Heterogeneity: Chi² = 0.80, df = 2 (P = 0.67); I² = 0%
Test for overall effect: Z = 10.49 (P < 0.00001)

Peto Odds Ratio Fixed, 95% CI — 0.01 0.1 1 10 100 — Less cough ARB   Less cough ACE-I

Outcome: Withdrawal due to adverse effects

Study or Subgroup	ARB Events	Total	ACE-I Events	Total	Weight	Peto Odds Ratio Fixed, 95% CI
Avanza 2000, cohort study	0	17	4	22	28.9%	0.15 [0.02, 1.14]
Verdeggia 2000, case-control	2	22	12	66	71.1%	0.51 [0.14, 1.90]
Total (95% CI)		**39**		**88**	**100.0%**	**0.36 [0.12, 1.08]**
Total events	2		16			

Heterogeneity: Chi² = 1.01, df = 1 (P = 0.31); I² = 1%
Test for overall effect: Z = 1.83 (P = 0.07)

Peto Odds Ratio Fixed, 95% CI — 0.01 0.1 1 10 100 — Less withdrawals ARB   Less withdrawals ACE-I

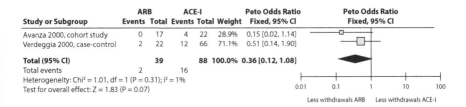

Review manager software is used to compute effects and produce Forest plots.

0.12 to 1.08 (Box C7.3). Such a large spread in the confidence interval indicated imprecision arising from a small number of participants and a low number of events.

Careful readers might have noticed in Box C7.3 that results from the cohort and the case-control study designs are combined. Study designs have different weaknesses and potentials for bias and should not normally be mixed up in meta-analysis. There is agreement that the results from randomized trials and observational studies should not be pooled. How best to synthesize non-randomized studies of different designs (e.g. cohort and case-control studies) is an issue of ongoing debate. It is clear that pooling does not compensate for methodological weaknesses.

Step 5: Interpreting the findings

How can we bring together what we have learnt in the previous Steps to come up with a decision? Step 1 has ranked the outcomes of interest according to their importance for patients. In Step 2, studies have been selected taking study design into consideration. Step 3 has reviewed the methodological quality of the selected observational studies. Step 4 has explored the heterogeneity of results and produced summary effects.

The gauging of the strength of the evidence is shown separately for each *outcome*, cough and withdrawal due to adverse effects, considering the observational data only (Box C7.4). For the *outcome* cough, the point estimate of OR showed an association. The 95% confidence interval around this estimate was very precise. In the absence of other features that impair the strength of the overall evidence, such a large effect could increase our

The Grading of Recommendations Assessment, Development and Evaluation (**GRADE**) working group is an informal collaboration aiming to develop a comprehensive methodology for assessing the strength of the evidence collated in systematic reviews and for generating recommendations from evidence in guidelines (gradeworkinggroup. org). Interpretation of findings in this case study draws on this methodology.

Box C7.4 Assessment of the strength of evidence for the outcomes cough and withdrawal due to adverse effects in observational studies comparing angiotensin-receptor blockers (ARBs) *versus* angiotensin-converting-enzyme inhibitors (ACE-Is)

Summary of results of observational studies

Importance of outcome	Outcome	Number of patients		Summary odds ratio, 95% confidence interval [CI] (heterogeneity)
		ARB	ACE-I	
Important	Cough			0.40
	3 observational studies	14,628	37,280	95% CI 0.34–0.48
	Total events: 691			(I^2 0%)
	Withdrawals			0.36
	2 observational studies	39	88	95% CI 0.12–1.08
	Total events: 18			(I^2 1%)

See Box C7.3 for Forest plots.

Gauging the strength of observational evidence

Strength is initially assessed as low due to the observational study design. Methodological limitations relegate the level of strength of evidence to very low.

Outcome	Study design	Study quality (risk of bias)*	Size of effect+	Dose–response gradient	Strength of evidence$
Cough	2 prospective cohorts, 1 cross-sectional cohort	Serious limitations	Large and precise	Not available	*Low*
	Initially assigned a low strength level	*→ Relegation*	*→ Increase*	*→ No change*	
Withdrawals due to adverse effects	1 prospective cohort 1 case-control	Serious limitations	Imprecise	Not available	*Very low*
	Initially assigned a low strength level	*→ Relegation*	*→ No change*	*→ No change*	

* See Box C7.2.

+ The methodological weaknesses of the studies were so serious that raising the strength level of evidence on grounds of large effect was not justifiable.

*$ Raised to a **high** level after consideration of randomized evidence which offered precise effect estimates from high-quality studies.*

*See Box 5.1 for levels of strength of evidence: **A very low** level signifies that we are very uncertain about the estimate of the effect, whereas a **high** level signifies that further research is very unlikely to change our confidence in the estimate.*

confidence that ARBs 'truly' lower the risk of cough compared to ACE-Is. The strong association between *exposure* and *outcome* is one feature of a causal association (Case study 9). Some authorities recommend using an OR value smaller than 0.5 or larger than 2 to define a strong association or large effect. Although observational studies are susceptible to bias and confounding that lead often to overestimation of the effects, it is unlikely that imbalance of prognostic factors between comparison groups will be solely responsible for very large effects. Additionally, the data reported in the review on cough from 37 randomized trials (not shown in this Case study) indicated a strong effect resulting in less cough for patients treated with ARBs.

Concerning withdrawals due to adverse effects, both studies reported fewer withdrawals for patients treated with ARBs compared to ACE-Is, but the estimation of association was imprecise. When assigning a level of strength to the evidence, the starting point is the study design. The lack of randomized treatment allocation makes observational studies start at a low strength level. Methodological limitations of included studies relegate the strength to a very low level. In this situation, even large effects

Strength of evidence describes the extent to which we can be confident that the estimate of an observed effect is correct for important questions. It takes into account the importance and directness of outcome measure, study design, study quality (risk of bias), heterogeneity, imprecision (confidence interval width) and publication bias (this is not an exhaustive list).

cannot justifiably raise the strength level. However, the data reported in the review on withdrawals due to adverse effects from 34 randomized trials (not shown in this Case study) indicated a strong effect resulting in fewer withdrawals for patients treated with ARBs. Considering this information, the strength level assigned to the overall evidence based on observational and experimental studies together was raised to high.

Resolution of scenario

The review as a whole, including evidence from both observational and randomized studies, reported with high strength of evidence that ACE-Is cause a higher frequency of cough than do ARBs in patients with hypertension. In addition, more patients on ACE-Is withdrew from the clinical trials due to adverse effects than patients on ARBs. Both drugs were known to have similar effectiveness in controlling blood pressure. For the decision-making, some other arguments outlined in Box 5.5 may be considered as well, e.g. availability and prices of the two alternatives and in some healthcare systems the co-payment by healthcare insurance. Since cough is fully reversible after stopping the ACE-Is, the patient, in order to reduce cost, may prefer to take the risk of adverse effects on ACE-Is first. Using the same evidence, another patient with different preferences may make a different, but informed, decision.

Case study 8:
Review of clinical practice guidelines

Luciano Mignini

Nationally, regionally and around the world, health professionals increasingly understand that healthcare must be based on scientific evidence, with knowledge synthesized in systematic reviews. Clinical practice guidelines underpinned by such reviews take the evidence forward when their recommendations are generated via a transparent process. Well-developed guidelines can be used to reduce inappropriate variations in practice and to promote the delivery of high-quality, evidence-based healthcare. They may also provide a mechanism by which healthcare professionals can be made accountable for clinical activities.

Healthcare professionals consult clinical practice guidelines to help them make decisions. Examples include deciding whether to order a test, to prescribe or change the dose of a drug or to refer a patient to a specialist. This Case study describes how clinical practice guidelines technically assemble evidence and systematically develop statements to assist practitioners in decision-making about appropriate healthcare for specific clinical circumstances.

Scenario: Screening for breast cancer

A 51-year-old woman without risk factors for breast cancer booked a clinic appointment seeking a clinical breast examination for breast cancer screening in your general practice. In this case, given the absence of risk factors, did clinical breast examination have a role? You wondered whether what sounded like a reasonable request was in fact in the woman's best interest. Might mammography not be the better screening option? The ages to start mammography, screening intervals and time to discontinue have been points of disagreement among your colleagues. You took the opportunity to review the recommended strategies for breast cancer screening in average-risk women.

What is involved in a clinical practice guideline?
Framing questions
↓
Identifying relevant reviews or conducting new reviews
↓
Assessing the quality of the reviews included and their evidence
↓
Summarizing the evidence to compare the benefits and harms of alternative care options
↓
Interpreting the finding, gauging the strength of evidence and making recommendations

Clinical practice guidelines or just **Guidelines** are systematically developed statements that include recommendations to assist practitioners and patients in making decisions about specific clinical situations. Ideally, they should use evidence from **systematic reviews** with an assessment of the benefits and harms of alternative care options.

Free-form question: It describes the query for which you seek an answer through a review in simple language (however vague).

Structured question: Reviewers convert free-form questions into a clear and explicit format using a structured approach (see Box 1.2). This makes the query potentially answerable through existing relevant studies.

DOI: 10.1201/9781003220039-15

Step 1: Framing the question

Free-form question

For asymptomatic women with an average risk for breast cancer, what is the best screening method among clinical breast examination and mammography?

Structured question

The participants	Asymptomatic women with average risk for breast cancer.
The interventions	Breast cancer screening methods: Clinical breast examination and mammography.
The outcomes	Mortality and morbidity.
The study design	Clinical practice guidelines.

Breast cancer is the most common cancer type in women and the fourth leading cause of cancer death. The evidence of interest to you is that which targets women without high risk. Absence of a personal history of breast cancer or high-risk breast lesions, absence of breast cancer-related genetic mutations (such as BRCA1/2 gene mutation or another familial breast cancer syndrome) and lack of history of exposure to radiation therapy to the chest in childhood are all part of defining average risk.

Step 2: Identifying relevant clinical practice guidelines

There are >6000 guidelines from 96 groups in 76 countries in the Guidelines International Network (g-i-n.net) database alone (Box 0.1). These days, everyone seems to be producing practice guidelines; sources include professional bodies, disease advocacy groups, government agencies and public and private health insurance organizations. This multiplicity of clinical practice guidelines creates a difficulty in determining which guidelines are trustworthy and which will be most likely to help in your practice presents. This Case study addresses this challenge.

Trip search for guidelines

Having framed your question, you decide to search Tripdatabase®. Trip or Turning Research Into Practice (tripdatabase.com) is a clinical search engine designed to allow users to quickly and easily find high-quality research evidence to support their practice. Trip has been online since 1997 and in that time has developed into one of the Internet's premier sources for evidence-based content. The Trip database may serve like any other search engine for medical research – plug-in your keywords into the box, press enter and watch what comes back. What makes Trip

---

Question components

The participants: A clinically suitable sample of patients.

The interventions: Comparison of groups with and without the intervention.

The outcomes: Changes in health status due to interventions.

The study design: Ways of conducting research to assess the effects of interventions.

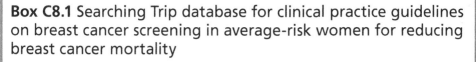

Box C8.1 Searching Trip database for clinical practice guidelines on breast cancer screening in average-risk women for reducing breast cancer mortality

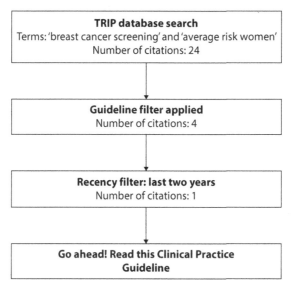

*The guideline is available at: Ann Intern Med 2019; **170**: 547–60, doi:10.7326/M18-2147.*

different is that it offers a guidelines filter – just click the guidelines button on the results page and only clinical practice guidelines appear on the screen. Importantly, Trip features an advanced search, including the ability to define the proximity of keywords within the structured question format. This is a fantastically logical way of translating your question into a search quickly.

You search Trip in structured question format by typing 'average-risk women' in the *participant* box and 'screening breast cancer' in the *intervention* box. By clicking the search button, and limiting the search to guidelines in the last 2 years (Box C8.1), you select the most updated guideline:

- Screening for Breast Cancer in average-risk women: A Guidance Statement from the American College of Physicians. *Ann Intern Med* 2019; **170**: 547–60, doi: 10.7326/M18-2147.

It reviewed all recent national guidelines on breast cancer screening in the Guidelines International Network library (Box 0.1) having checked for updates till 2018, the year before publication. In this sense, it is an umbrella review collating existing guidelines. In total, seven guidelines covering the time period from 2014 to 2018 are reviewed.

Step 3: Assessing the quality of the selected guideline

Clinical practice guidelines contain recommendations to help in the care of individual patients and also to establish practice standards. Physicians' confidence in guidelines has to be based on the assessment of its rigour. Ideally, there should be an objective process for developing recommendations based on a systematic review of evidence comparing the benefits and harms of alternative care options. The guideline group should comprise multidisciplinary experts including patient representatives who bring in the expertise gained through the lived experience of an illness. The group membership should have been screened for potential biases and conflicts of interests. Poor-quality guidelines are unlikely to help patient care. Good-quality guidelines provide the fundamental evidence base for improving clinical outcomes. In addition, because evidence generation is dynamic, guidelines should be updated frequently. This is why you chose the most updated guideline on breast cancer screening in this Case study.

This guideline collated seven others published before it, making its methodology akin to umbrella reviews (Case study 1). For its quality assessment, a two-step approach is required: First, an assessment of its own overall quality and then an assessment of the quality of the individual included guidelines. The AGREE II (Appraisal of Guidelines for REsearch and Evaluation, version II) is a set of validated tools for evaluating the quality and reporting of guidelines. An additional purpose of AGREE II is to provide a methodological strategy for the development of guidelines. The checklist includes specific assessment questions that cover many aspects of the quality of guidelines with a focus on methodological rigour. To capture the comprehensiveness, completeness, and transparency of reporting in a guideline, it consists of 23 appraisal criteria or items grouped in six independent quality domains: scope and purpose; stakeholder involvement; rigour of development; clarity of presentation; applicability; and editorial independence. Additionally, there are two overall assessment items: one to evaluate the overall guideline quality and the other to judge whether the guideline should be recommended for use in practice. When applying AGREE II, a score is assigned to each item. The higher the score, the more the quality criteria met. Each of the AGREE II items and the two global rating items are rated on a 7-point scale (1 – strongly disagree to 7 – strongly agree).

Your guideline scores well in each domain and overall (Box C8.2). How about the quality of the guidelines included? Four of the seven scored >5 in the overall assessment, and the other three scored low. Hence, you would have to look carefully at how the evidence was synthesized (Step 4) and interpreted (Step 5) and be very cautious when drawing your own conclusion.

An **umbrella review** is an evidence synthesis in the form of an overview of systematic reviews on a topic. Following a critical appraisal of all the relevant reviews, it aims to provide underpinning evidence for evidence-based practice.

Effect is a measure of association between an *intervention* and an *outcome*.

The **precision of effect** relates to the degree of uncertainty in the estimation of effect that is due to the play of chance. The confidence interval tells us about precision. The wider the confidence interval, the lower is the precision of the estimate of the effect.

Box C8.2 Assessing the quality of a clinical practice guideline concerning breast cancer screening using AGREE II checklist

Guideline quality domains	Guideline score*
1. Scope and purpose (the overall aim of the guideline)	7
2. Stakeholder involvement (role and expectations of stakeholders)	6
3. Rigour of development (gathering and summarizing the evidence)	6
4. Clarity of presentation (technical guidance)	6
5. Applicability (barriers and facilitators to implementation)	6
6. Editorial independence (identifying potential biases)	6
Overall guideline assessment	**6**

* Each of the AGREE II domains and items within it including the two global rating items for overall score is rated on a 7-point scale (1 – strongly disagree to 7 – strongly agree). A score of 1 is given when there is no information that is relevant to the AGREE II item, if the concept is very poorly reported or if the authors state explicitly that criteria were not met. A score of 7 is given if the quality of reporting is exceptional and where the full criteria and considerations given in the user's manual have been met.

AGREE II is available from agreetrust.org/agree-ii.

*The guideline assessed is available at: Ann Intern Med 2019; **170**: 547–60, doi: 10.1210/clinem/dgab742.*

Step 4: Summarizing the evidence

The goal of breast cancer screening is to gain benefit in terms of mortality, both specific to breast cancer and overall, with acceptable trade-offs against harmful outcomes such as overdiagnosis, overtreatment resulting from false positive test results, etc. The guideline synthesized the evidence as follows: Concerning clinical breast examination, the guideline said that while this may be seen as a screening option in low-resource settings, no studies had in fact shown any clinical benefit. The guideline concluded that it contributed no significant reduction in breast cancer mortality, considering the result of one randomized trial. Additionally, it noted that the harm associated with clinical breast examination was false positive results which in turn would inevitably cause undue morbidity. Thus, it is blatantly recommended against clinical breast examination.

Turning to mammography, the guideline showed that although evidence could not demonstrate an effect on overall mortality, there was a reduction in the relative risk for breast cancer mortality for women aged 50 to 69 years in randomized trials. In this subgroup, there were precise, statistically significant, results for the outcome breast cancer mortality (one of the included guidelines provided a relative risk point estimate of 0.86 with a 95% confidence interval of 0.75–0.99). The guideline

Strength of evidence describes the extent to which we can be confident that the estimate of an observed effect is correct for critical and important *outcomes*. It takes into account the directness of outcome measure, study design, study quality, heterogeneity, imprecision of the effect and publication bias (this is not an exhaustive list).

considered experimental and observational evidence on harms including overdiagnosis, overtreatment and other test-related inconveniences and adverse effects. It then weighed up the benefits *versus* harms.

Step 5: Interpreting the findings

This clinical practice guideline undertook a review of the evidence contained in seven existing guidelines to generate its own recommendations. In doing so, it weighed the evidence considering the importance of outcomes, it balanced the various screening options for their benefits *versus* harms and it looked for consensus among the guidelines it captured. Although it did not deploy the GRADE methodology explicitly, it did implicitly gauge the strength of the evidence as part of its process leading to its recommendations. In addition, it provided the data on relative risks and computed information on numbers needed to treat in its appendices. It appeared that all the ingredients for making rational recommendations were there. It balanced desirable *versus* undesirable effects, taking the strength of evidence into account (Box 5.5).

Of particular interest to your case was the subgroup analyses for women aged 50–69 years. The guideline's recommendation concerning clinical breast examination was negative: 'In average-risk women of all ages, clinicians should not use clinical breast examination to screen for breast cancer'. Its recommendation concerning mammography was positive: 'In average-risk women aged 50 to 74 years, clinicians should offer screening for breast cancer with biennial mammography'. In addition, there was a recommendation about the cessation of screening: 'In average-risk women aged 75 years or older or in women with a life expectancy of 10 years or less, clinicians should discontinue screening for breast cancer'.

What remains is for you to gauge the patient's values and preferences in light of her initial request for a clinical breast examination.

The Grading of Recommendations Assessment, Development and Evaluation (**GRADE**) working group is an informal collaboration that aims to develop a comprehensive methodology for assessing the strength of the evidence collated in systematic reviews and for generating recommendations from evidence in guidelines (gradeworkinggroup. org).

Resolution of scenario

Your 51-year-old woman without risk factors has booked an appointment requesting screening for breast cancer via clinical breast examination. In recent discussions, your colleagues had expressed doubts about mammography as a screening test in low-risk women. You now have a high-quality clinical practice guideline in hand. It addresses the questions about ages to start and discontinue mammography, screening intervals and the role of both clinical breast examination and mammography. Having considered the information provided in the guideline, and knowing that advancing age itself is a risk factor for breast cancer, you are confident to decline her request for screening with clinical breast examination alone. You recommend screening for breast cancer with biennial mammography to your patient. You decide to share the guideline with her making a short presentation about your understanding of the evidence contained in it in lay terms. She can now read it in anticipation of accepting your advice and has the opportunity to return to you if she has questions.

Case study 9: *Systematic reviews to assess a prognostic factor*

Systematic reviews commonly address questions about the effectiveness of therapy and the accuracy of testing. However, evidence also needs to be summarized to increase our understanding of aetiology and prognosis. It is, therefore, logical to expect that systematic reviews need to be performed to synthesize research into these areas. Typically, comparative observational studies relate the effect of various *exposures* on *outcomes* to inform questions about aetiology and prognosis. Because observational studies are prone to the influence of confounding, it is not always certain if the relationships between observed *exposures* and *outcomes* in these studies are likely to be causal.

Many studies try to identify prognostic factors for *outcomes* after diagnosis of disease. A prognostic factor is any measure taken from clinical history, examination or tests that is associated with subsequent clinical *outcome*. Prognostic factors help distinguish groups of patients with a different, worse, or better than average, prognosis. This information can be used to provide targeted care. The individual studies that investigate prognostic factors frequently show inconsistent findings and systematic reviews offer an avenue for the objective evaluation of the prognostic value of a given factor. They seek, through meta-analysis, to verify whether a potential prognostic factor is associated with the *outcome* and to estimate the strength of the association. The observed relationship between prognostic factor and *outcome* may also be assessed for the possibility of there being a causal association in such reviews.

This Case study describes the basics of how to evaluate a prognostic factor and how to apply the criteria for a causal association through a systematic review. These steps are illustrated using a published review concerning the hypothesized relationship of obesity as a prognostic factor after a prostate cancer diagnosis.

Scenario: Is obesity a prognostic factor for survival after a prostate cancer diagnosis?

In men, prostate cancer is a leading cause of death. As a general practitioner, you are aware that obesity is related to prostate cancer severity at the time of diagnosis. You have wondered if obesity is also a prognostic factor that reduces survival after the diagnosis has been made. Weight is modifiable through lifestyle changes, so you are keen to know if you can offer something positive to your prostate cancer patients. You look for

Step 1
Framing questions

↓

Step 2
Identifying relevant literature

↓

Step 3
Assessing the quality of the literature

↓

Step 4
Summarizing the evidence

↓

Step 5
Interpreting the findings

Confounding is a situation in comparative studies where the effect of an *exposure* on an *outcome* is distorted due to the association of the *outcome* with another factor, which can prevent or cause the *outcome* independent of the *exposure* and it is associated with the *exposure*. Data analysis may be adjusted for confounding in observational studies.

Prognosis is a probable course or *outcome* of a disease. **Prognostic factors** are patient or disease characteristics that influence the *outcome*. A good prognosis is associated with a low rate of undesirable outcomes. A poor prognosis is associated with a high rate of undesirable outcomes.

DOI: 10.1201/9781003220039-16

an evidence synthesis on the association between obesity and prostate cancer mortality. You search PubMed from the sources of reviews shown in Box 0.1. Typing the words 'obesity' AND 'prostate cancer mortality' in the query box and clicking the search button, there are 132 hits. You apply the systematic review filter in the above PubMed search and get just 13 citations. Reading through titles and abstracts ordered according to date of publication, you find the following review in the first position:

- Obesity as a risk factor for prostate cancer mortality: A systematic review and dose–response meta-analysis of 280,199 patients. *Cancers* 2021; **13**: 4169, doi: 10.3390/cancers13164169.

It is suitable for addressing your question about prognosis. It also appears to be suitable for evaluating a causal association as the title indicates an attempt to examine one of the causal criteria, i.e. dose–response relationship.

Step 1: Framing the question

Free-form question

Among patients diagnosed with prostate cancer, is obesity a prognostic factor causing a reduction in survival?

Structured questions

The participants	People with prostate cancer diagnosed.
The exposures	Obesity *versus* healthy weight. Obesity as a prognostic factor can be measured in many different ways, e.g. weight in kg as a continuous variable or categories of weight/height^2 or BMI, the body mass index. In this Case study, we present the findings of the analysis using two *exposure* categories: obese BMI >30 and healthy weight BMI <25. In addition, other prognostic factors, e.g. disease stage at the time to diagnosis, etc., may have an influence on the *outcome* simultaneously.
The outcomes	Prostate cancer mortality.
The study designs	Observational comparative studies (Box 1.4). Cohort studies permit temporal evaluation of the relationship between exposure and outcome. Multivariable analyses adjust for the simultaneous effect of *exposures* other than obesity.

Having framed the structured question, let's look at how a systematic review can synthesize the findings to evaluate a prognostic factor.

Free-form question: It describes the query for which you seek an answer through a review in simple language (however vague).

Structured question: Reviewers convert free-form questions into a clear and explicit format using a structured approach (see Box 1.2). This makes the query potentially answerable through existing relevant studies.

Causal association criteria evaluable via a systematic review include amongst others: temporality, consistency, strength, dose–response relationship and biological plausibility of the association observed across included studies of acceptable quality.

Question components

The participants: A clinically suitable sample of patients.

The interventions: Comparison of groups with and without the exposure.

The outcomes: Changes in health status due to exposure.

The study design: Ways of conducting research to assess the effects of exposure.

The evaluation of causal criteria helps us to undertake an assessment of whether the association observed between *exposure* to the prognostic factor and *outcome* is likely to be due to a causal link, not just a statistical association. Some of the key criteria evaluable via a systematic review with meta-analysis include: temporality, consistency, strength and dose–response relationship of the association observed across included studies. There should also be biological plausibility with a suggested mechanism. We will cover each of these criteria within the Steps below.

> **Effect** is a measure of association between an *exposure* and an *outcome*. In this Case study, the **hazard ratio** measured the effect by comparing the survival experience of the *exposure* groups. The size of the effect is a measure of the strength criteria for the assessment of causal association.

Step 2: Identifying relevant literature

Multiple sources were searched using an appropriate search term combination adapted for each database to yield as many relevant citations as possible of primary studies that evaluated the association between obesity and prostate cancer mortality. There were no language restrictions and reference lists were also scrutinized to identify any studies not captured by the electronic searches. Of the 7278 citations initially identified, 107 were submitted to a detailed eligibility assessment, and a total of 57 published articles were included (Box C9.1). Of these, 37 provided comparative data on the association of the prognostic factor categorized as obese BMI ≥30 and healthy weight BMI <25 with prostate cancer mortality. There were 245,279 *participants* with 20,721 *outcome* events in these studies in total.

Step 3: Assessing study quality

Study design threshold for study selection

The comparative observational *design* served as the threshold for study selection to ensure that studies without data on outcomes of participants of healthy weight were excluded. The *design*-based selection criterion permitted the inclusion of both cohort and case-control studies. Here it is important to highlight that cohort studies are considered the preferred *design* for evaluating a prognostic factor and a causal association (Box 1.4, 4.2). This is because it provides data that is temporal in nature, i.e. *exposure* is ascertained first and then, after follow-up over a period of time, *outcome* is measured. The association of *exposure* with *outcome* is measured as the frequency of *outcome* within *exposure* groups being compared. Thus, the temporal association criterion for a causal association is readily satisfied in cohort studies. By contrast, case-control studies do not follow a temporal sequence naturally in the *design*. In this *design*, *outcome* measurement is the starting point, and *exposure* ascertainment happens via a retrospective process that is subject to various

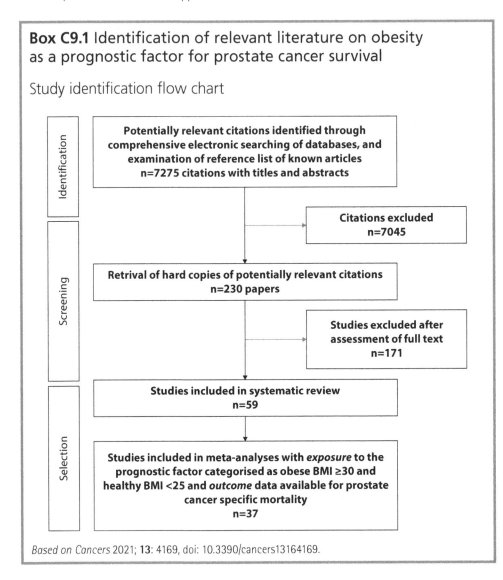

Box C9.1 Identification of relevant literature on obesity as a prognostic factor for prostate cancer survival

Study identification flow chart

Based on Cancers 2021; **13**: 4169, doi: 10.3390/cancers13164169.

forms of biases. Thus, case-control studies measure the association by comparing the odds of *exposure* in groups with and without *outcome*.

Quality assessment of comparative observational studies

In order for the measured effects to represent a valid estimate of the association, the included studies should have sought to minimize biases and errors in their study protocol, as well as in study conduct and analysis. In this review, a detailed quality assessment checklist, the Newcastle-Ottawa

The **validity** of a study depends on the degree to which its design, conduct and analysis minimize **biases**.

scale, was used to capture the risk of bias after appropriate customization to take into account the clinical components of the question. Around two-thirds of the studies were of high-moderate quality (Box C9.2).

It is important to extract and capture the features that will permit statistical synthesis to evaluate the association of the prognostic factor with the *outcome* and whether the association meets causal criteria. Prospective cohort studies readily meet the temporal association criterion for establishing causality. The ascertainment of *exposure* should happen via secure records unbiased by preoccupation about the

> **Bias** either exaggerates or underestimates the 'true' effect of an *exposure*.

Box C9.2 Study design and quality features relevant for the assessment of the risk of bias in observational studies evaluating obesity as a prognostic factor for prostate cancer survival

Study design

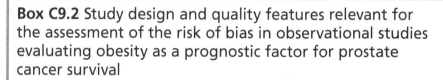
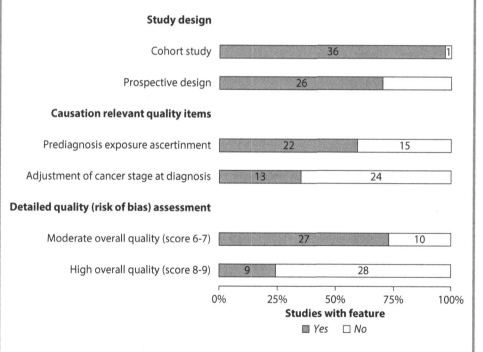

	Yes	No

Study design
- Cohort study: 36 | 1
- Prospective design: 26

Causation relevant quality items
- Prediagnosis exposure ascertinment: 22 | 15
- Adjustment of cancer stage at diagnosis: 13 | 24

Detailed quality (risk of bias) assessment
- Moderate overall quality (score 6-7): 27 | 10
- High overall quality (score 8-9): 9 | 28

0%   25%   50%   75%   100%
Studies with feature
■ Yes   □ No

*Based on Cancers 2021; **13**: 4169, doi: 10.3390/cancers13164169.*

Information is presented as 100% stacked bars. Data in the stacks represent a number of studies.

*Study quality (risk of bias) was assessed and scored using the Newcastle-Ottawa Scale (NOS), a generic checklist for comparative observational studies. NOS scoring ranges from 0 to 9, with <6 being low overall quality (ohri.ca/Programs/clinical_epidemiology/oxford.asp). Another tool for QUality In Prognosis Studies is called QUIPS (Ann Intern Med 2013; **158**: 280–6, doi: 10.7326/0003-4819-158-4-201302190-00009).*

premature occurrence of *outcome* and unaffected by the course of disease following diagnosis, e.g. measurement of height and weight before the diagnosis of prostate cancer. The comparability of *exposure* groups should be ensured or data should be collected on other important prognostic variable(s) for making statistical adjustments for confounding in the analysis, e.g. cancer stage at the time of diagnosis is bound to be associated with the *outcome* independent of the obesity *exposure*. Data analysis may be adjusted for confounding by using multivariable models in observational studies. In addition to these individual items, which are part of the generic quality checklists, the overall quality of the studies themselves is an important feature for the valid assessment of causal association.

Heterogeneity is the variation of effects between studies. It may arise because of differences between studies in key characteristics of their *participants, exposures* and *outcomes* (clinical heterogeneity), and their *study designs* and quality (methodological heterogeneity).

Step 4: Summarizing the evidence

The overall meta-analysis shows an association between *exposure* to obesity as a prognostic factor (obese = BMI ≥30 *versus* healthy weight = BMI <25) and prostate cancer mortality (Box C9.3).

Causal criteria for which data synthesis examined the association between *exposure* to obesity and prostate cancer mortality included temporality, strength and consistency of association. The temporality of the association between *exposure* to obesity and prostate cancer mortality is correctly verified by the use of cohort study design, especially in the subgroup of prospective studies. For the strength of association, we can combine individual study results in the meta-analysis (Box C9.3). Look at the summary estimate of the hazard ratio which shows a 19% mortality among obese patients compared to those with a healthy weight. This point estimate may vary and considering the 95% confidence interval, the certainty level in the estimation ranges from 10% to 28%. The 95% confidence intervals are a means of capturing the likelihood of the play of chance in the result obtained. It is conventional to describe the result as significant if the 95% confidence interval does not include the value 1.0 of the effect measured.

The consistency causal criterion refers to the repeated observation of the association in different populations under different circumstances. Whether the association varies across studies is examined by the evaluation of heterogeneity, by visual inspection of Forest plots and statistically (Box C9.3). The majority of the studies, 30 of 37 to be exact, have a point estimate of the hazard ratio above the value of 1.0, i.e. consistent with the possibility of there being a relationship between obesity and prostate cancer mortality. The overall statistical level of inconsistency is moderate with an I^2 of 44%. I^2 range lies between 0% and 100%; the value of 0% indicates no observed heterogeneity and larger values show increasing heterogeneity. Graphical representations aid in the exploration of consistency. It becomes obvious that heterogeneity is arising from studies with variation in the size of the relationship between obesity and increased prostate cancer mortality, not from studies without a relationship (there are only

Box C9.3 Meta-analysis of studies examining the association between *exposure* to obesity (BMI ≥30 *versus* BMI <25) and prostate cancer mortality

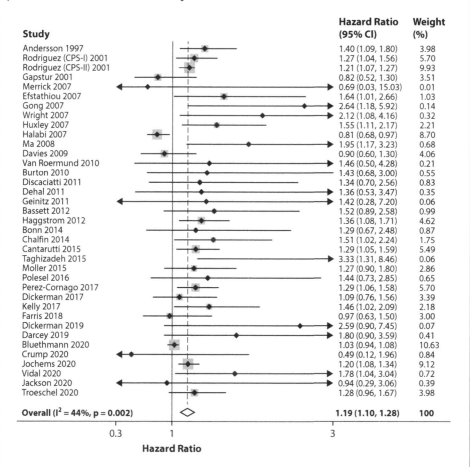

Study	Hazard Ratio (95% CI)	Weight (%)
Andersson 1997	1.40 (1.09, 1.80)	3.98
Rodriguez (CPS-I) 2001	1.27 (1.04, 1.56)	5.70
Rodriguez (CPS-II) 2001	1.21 (1.07, 1.27)	9.93
Gapstur 2001	0.82 (0.52, 1.30)	3.51
Merrick 2007	0.69 (0.03, 15.03)	0.01
Efstathiou 2007	1.64 (1.01, 2.66)	1.03
Gong 2007	2.64 (1.18, 5.92)	0.14
Wright 2007	2.12 (1.08, 4.16)	0.32
Huxley 2007	1.55 (1.11, 2.17)	2.21
Halabi 2007	0.81 (0.68, 0.97)	8.70
Ma 2008	1.95 (1.17, 3.23)	0.68
Davies 2009	0.90 (0.60, 1.30)	4.06
Van Roermund 2010	1.46 (0.50, 4.28)	0.21
Burton 2010	1.43 (0.68, 3.00)	0.55
Discaciatti 2011	1.34 (0.70, 2.56)	0.83
Dehal 2011	1.36 (0.53, 3.47)	0.35
Geinitz 2011	1.42 (0.28, 7.20)	0.06
Bassett 2012	1.52 (0.89, 2.58)	0.99
Haggstrom 2012	1.36 (1.08, 1.71)	4.62
Bonn 2014	1.29 (0.67, 2.48)	0.87
Chalfin 2014	1.51 (1.02, 2.24)	1.75
Cantarutti 2015	1.29 (1.05, 1.59)	5.49
Taghizadeh 2015	3.33 (1.31, 8.46)	0.06
Moller 2015	1.27 (0.90, 1.80)	2.86
Polesel 2016	1.44 (0.73, 2.85)	0.65
Perez-Cornago 2017	1.29 (1.06, 1.58)	5.70
Dickerman 2017	1.09 (0.76, 1.56)	3.39
Kelly 2017	1.46 (1.02, 2.09)	2.18
Farris 2018	0.97 (0.63, 1.50)	3.00
Dickerman 2019	2.59 (0.90, 7.45)	0.07
Darcey 2019	1.80 (0.90, 3.59)	0.41
Bluethmann 2020	1.03 (0.94, 1.08)	10.63
Crump 2020	0.49 (0.12, 1.96)	0.84
Jochems 2020	1.20 (1.08, 1.34)	9.12
Vidal 2020	1.78 (1.04, 3.04)	0.72
Jackson 2020	0.94 (0.29, 3.06)	0.39
Troeschel 2020	1.28 (0.96, 1.67)	3.98
Overall (I^2 = 44%, p = 0.002)	**1.19 (1.10, 1.28)**	**100**

Hazard Ratio (0.3 — 1 — 3)

*Based on Cancers 2021; **13**: 4169, doi: 10.3390/cancers13164169.*

Random effects model was used for meta-analysis (see Boxes 4.3. and 4.4).

Hazard ratio >1 indicates increased prostate cancer mortality among obese patients compared to those with a healthy weight.

seven studies with point estimates of hazard ratio <1.0 and only one of these is statistically significant). The key to understanding the impact of the inconsistency lies in evaluating the studies' characteristics. The table in Box C9.4 with its subgroup meta-analyses shows the differences between the studies at a glance. The studies subgrouped by good design and quality (quality items and overall risk of bias) features show consistent association across the meta-analyses.

Box C9.4 Data synthesis to evaluate casual criteria in the meta-analysis of studies examining the association between exposure to obesity (BMI ≥30 *versus* BMI <25) and prostate cancer mortality

Causal criteria	Meta-analysis group (number of studies)	Association (summary hazard ratio)	95% Confidence interval	Inconsistency I^2
Temporal association Prospective cohort studies permit the assessment of temporality	• Cohort studies (n = 36)	1.19	1.11–1.28	46%
	• Prospective design (n = 26)	1.19	1.10–1.28	34%
Strong and consistent association The overall meta-analytic summary effect and the estimation of heterogeneity, respectively, permit the assessment of the strength and consistency of the association	• Overall (n = 37)	1.19	1.10–1.28	44%
Valid estimation of the association Correct exposure ascertainment and adjustment for confounding are key quality items for risk of bias assessment	• Pre-diagnosis BMI (n = 22)	1.23	1.17–1.30	0%
	• Adjustment for cancer stage at diagnosis (n = 13)	1.11	0.95–1.27	44%
Calculation of a quality score can be used to evaluate the overall risk of bias	• *High-quality score (n = 9)	1.24	1.14–1.35	0%
	• *Moderate quality score (n = 27)	1.17	1.07–1.27	49%
Biological gradient Dose–response relationship evaluates if higher levels of exposure are associated with poorer outcomes. For this analysis, the exposure variable has been changed to a continuous scale.	• BMI exposure on continuous scale (unit 5 kg/m²) (n = 31)	1.09	1.05–1.12	44%

* Study quality (risk of bias) assessed and scored using the Newcastle–Ottawa Scale (NOS), a generic checklist for observational studies. NOS scoring ranges from 0 to 9, with <6 being low overall quality (ohri.ca/Programs/clinical_epidemiology/oxford.asp).

Based on Cancers 2021; 13: 4169, doi: 10.3390/cancers13164169.

Dose–response relationship or biological gradient is another causal criterion for which the exposure variable would need to be changed to a continuous scale. There were 31 studies where BMI *exposure* was reported on a continuous scale (unit 5 kg/m^2), so it was feasible to examine if higher levels of exposure are associated with poorer survival (Box C9.4). Meta-analysis using continuous *exposure* measurement showed that with rising BMI (per 5 kg/m^2 units) there was on average a 9% increase in prostate cancer mortality.

Step 5: Interpreting the findings

Is obesity a prognostic factor for prostate cancer survival? There is certainly an association in the overall meta-analysis. How far did the association satisfy causal criteria? In evaluating causal criteria, there is no accepted scoring system to decide whether there is sufficient evidence of a causal association. In fact, it can be safely said that all such assessments at best produce a tentative conclusion. Formal examination of individual hypotheses concerning temporality, consistency, strength, dose–response relationship and the biological plausibility of suggested mechanisms can be employed to assess causality, tentatively.

As shown in Box C9.4, in studies with temporality and quality, the observed association was moderately strong with some inconsistency. A dose–response association was found regarding higher levels of *exposure* and prostate cancer specific mortality. These findings appeared to hold when all-cause mortality was used as the *outcome* measure, lending credence to the causal association hypotheses. The inferences concerning mechanisms of the disease need to be carefully generated and are best done via a systematic review of the related basic research. The discussion section of the review commented on biological plausibility and coherence stating that there were analogous causal relationships between obesity and mortality in other cancers too. Thus, the observed association of higher BMI levels with increased mortality in prostate cancer, after cautious interpretation, appears to be causally linked.

Resolution of the scenario

After having read, and hopefully understood, the review, you know more about the suggested role of obesity as a modifiable prognostic factor in prostate cancer survival. This review supports the theory that obesity is potentially causally linked to prostate cancer mortality. It has, therefore, highlighted the need for considering lifestyle interventions to control weight in prostate cancer patients.

Case study 10:
Publishing systematic reviews: Tips and tricks for convincing journal editors and peer reviewers

Step 1
Framing questions
↓
Step 2
Identifying relevant literature
↓
Step 3
Assessing the quality of the literature
↓
Step 4
Summarizing the evidence
↓
Step 5
Interpreting the findings

New reviewers find it difficult to navigate the process of publication for their drafted manuscripts. They lack knowledge about the journals' assessments, which makes it hard to get their reviews accepted on the first submission. Even experienced reviewers frequently face rejection by journal editors. Time is wasted in the rejection–resubmission cycle. The purpose of this Case study is to familiarize new reviewers with the written and unwritten publication rules. With our extensive experience in editing, peer-reviewing, supervising, writing and rewriting, we share some tips and tricks for getting a review manuscript accepted. So, let's go!

This Case study is based on the real experience of a Master's degree student. It demonstrates how to convert a well-conducted systematic review into a succinct manuscript for submission as an article to a peer-reviewed journal. It will give an overview of the publication process and will provide guidance on drafting a convincing paper. Based on peer-review reports, journal editors will ask you to make revisions to your submitted paper before accepting it for publication (Box C10.1). They may of course not like the submission or peer-review reports may not be too encouraging, so the paper may be rejected. It may take several resubmissions before finally being accepted. This Case study will help avoid rejection by identifying the common pitfalls. On publication, the systematic review will be indexed in various online databases and its findings will become available to a wide audience.

Scenario: Having completed a Master's degree thesis you wish to have your literature review published as a journal article

You are a Master's degree student who has had the wisdom to undertake a systematic review for your thesis. The thesis is a voluminous document with an unstructured abstract and the main text has several chapters with a word count of 50,000. You are being encouraged to publish the literature review as a journal article. This will take effort as you will need

DOI: 10.1201/9781003220039-17

Box C10.1 Manuscript assessment in a peer-reviewed journal

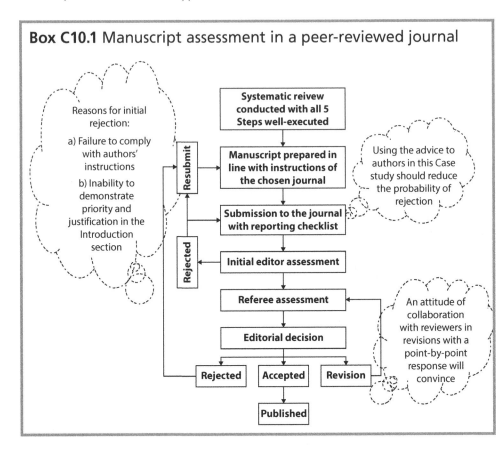

Reasons for initial rejection:

a) Failure to comply with authors' instructions

b) Inability to demonstrate priority and justification in the Introduction section

Systematic reivew conducted with all 5 Steps well-executed

Manuscript prepared in line with instructions of the chosen journal

Submission to the journal with reporting checklist

Initial editor assessment

Referee assessment

Editorial decision

Resubmit

Rejected

Rejected   Accepted   Revision

Published

Using the advice to authors in this Case study should reduce the probability of rejection

An attitude of collaboration with reviewers in revisions with a point-by-point response will convince

to abridge the thesis into a structured abstract and main text of around 3000 words. You feel that your literature review findings will not really get known without this additional effort. However, you don't even know where to start. Your tutors have little time to give you guidance or perhaps they have themselves not published much. Where do you go from here?

You have learnt all about the various Steps of a systematic review given in the first section of this book. You have applied them in conducting your own review and in writing it up as a Master's thesis according to the instructions of your University. Your written thesis has been assessed and passed by your examiners. You will soon be awarded the degree. The publication is an important personal and professional milestone for you. Your task now is to take the writing tips for systematic review authors given at the end of each Step in the first section of this book and abridge your thesis document into a manuscript according to the instructions of your chosen journal (Box C10.1). The journal may require you to provide a reporting checklist so you start to prepare one as you write.

As a reviewer, you would naturally base your work on previously published studies, so it is critical that your writing is free of plagiarism, something that most journals would automatically check for on receiving

Plagiarism: The act of presenting the text as your own that is an identical copy of the text that is previously published. Using artificial intelligence software programs such as CrossCheck or iThenticate, journals can look up within milliseconds text chunks that are copies of already published articles.

your submission. When taking data from included articles for your review, careful paraphrasing or quotation of the original text with reference to the source will be required to avoid allegations of scientific misconduct.

Step 1: Framing the question

Free-form question

Is there a gap in vaccination coverage among migrants compared to the local population?

Structured question

The population	People who need vaccination.
The exposures	Migrants compared to local or native-born people.
The outcome	Vaccination coverage.
The study design	Systematic review of controlled observational studies.

You have learned in your systematic review course, aided by this book, that prospective registration is an essential feature of a good review. When registering the topic for your Master's thesis, you had to think hard about the review question. Having framed the question, and before performing the literature searches, the first thing you've done is to go ahead and prospectively register your review:

- Vaccination coverage in migrants and non-migrants: A systematic review. *Prospero* 2021 CRD42021228061. www.crd.york.ac.uk/prospero/display_record.php?ID=CRD42021228061

The relevant reporting checklist given the observational design of the studies to be selected is MOOSE, a guideline for meta-analyses of observational studies in epidemiology. Regardless of whether your reporting checklist is MOOSE or PRISMA, we have to keep in mind that scientific articles follow a rigid structure.

The skeleton of the main manuscript text can be summarized according to the acronym IMRaD. All the parts of the submission are not equally important. As the saying goes, the first impression is the last impression! We know that title and abstract are read first and are, thus, key to convincing the editors and peer reviewers, so you should start writing these to begin with. We don't advise you to wait to write the main manuscript ahead of the abstract. Yes, this appears counterintuitive. Don't fear. Writing title and abstract first has always worked, and worked well, in the over 500 papers we have published between us as co-authors.

Free-form question: It describes the query for which you seek an answer through a review in simple language (however vague).

Structured question: Reviewers convert free-form questions into a clear and explicit format using a structured approach (Box 1.2). This makes the query potentially answerable through existing relevant studies.

IMRaD is an acronym that refers to the section headings used in writing the main manuscript text, i.e. I-Introduction, M-Methods, R-Results, a-and, D-Discussion, of a paper for submission to a peer-reviewed journal.

Reporting guidelines are checklists for writing manuscripts. They provide a list of reporting items with a flow diagram to enhance the transparency of the manuscript (see www.equator-network.org). Most journals require authors to submit a relevant systematic review reporting checklist (e.g. PRISMA, MOOSE, MARS, etc.). This assists peer-reviewers and editors in their assessment of compliance of the manuscript with good methodology and reporting standards.

Taking the advice from the writing tips at the end of Step 1 and the MOOSE checklist, you ensure that as many components of the structured question as possible are included in the succinct title (Box C10.2). In particular, the design element is included in the subtitle, making clear that the paper is about a systematic review with a meta-analysis. The title of the manuscript to be submitted to the journal is cognate with the prospectively registered title. If the registered title, the paper title and the objective statements in the abstract and the last paragraph of the introduction all consistently refer to your structured question, there is a good chance that the editors and peer reviewers will take you to be a serious reviewer who can be trusted.

Having got the title and the abstract right, you turn to the main text of the manuscript. In the introduction section of the main text, you ensure that the last paragraph covers the review's structured question when describing the objective. In the methods section, you provide the prospective registration details again. All of this sets you off on the correct footing. On initial editor assessment, the journal editor finds your article to be potentially publishable and sends it out to obtain peer review.

Abstract: Write it first! Draft it in a structured format to be a stand-alone text that can be understood completely on its own without the need to refer to the main text. Provide the prospective registration details. Stay within the permitted word limits. Keep returning to it to revise and improve it while drafting the main manuscript text.

Box C10.2 Relation between Step 1 of a systematic review and the title of its paper, its abstract and the introduction section of the main text

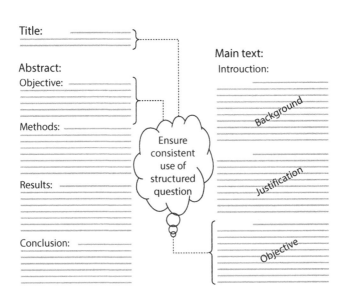

Example of consistent use of the elements of structured question in a paper:

Structured question:

The population	People who need vaccination.
The exposures	Migrants compared to local or native-born people.
The outcome	Vaccination coverage.
The study design	Systematic review of controlled observational studies.

Prospective registration of the review

Prospectively registered title: 'Vaccination coverage in migrants and non-migrants: A systematic review'

Title, Abstract and Introduction in the published paper

Title: 'Vaccination coverage among migrants: A systematic review and meta-analysis'.
Abstract – objective: 'This systematic review assessed quantitatively the level of vaccination coverage among migrants, in comparison with non-migrants, collating the published literature'.
Introduction – last paragraph: 'The objective of this systematic review was to quantitatively determine the level of vaccination coverage among migrants compared to non-migrants, collating the published observational studies'.

Based on *Semergen*, 2022; **48**: 96–105, doi: 10.1016/j.semerg.2021.10.008, and *Prospero* 2021 crd.york.ac.uk/prospero/display_record.php?ID=CRD42021228061

Step 2: Identifying relevant literature

You used Mendeley Reference Manager software for bibliographic management during literature search and selection. It also plugs into the word processing software for citing literature in the main manuscript text and generating a bibliography. This makes your writing task easier.

For writing the background and justification paragraphs of the introduction section of the manuscript (Box C10.2), there is an additional tip here: When you had started to register your review online, *Prospero* had asked you if you had searched to identify similar reviews? Using the sources listed in the Introduction chapter of this book (Box 0.1), you had checked to see if similar reviews already existed. These initial searches for reviews had determined that previous evidence syntheses were too narrowly focused geographically. This was an informal search that permitted you to register your review prospectively. Subsequently, in Step 2 of the review, when you formally searched and screened citations (Section 2.3.2) for studies that addressed your review question, you also ensured that you captured all previous systematic review citations on your topic. This allowed you to capture relevant references for drafting a strong background and justification for your paper. Getting this right is one of the keys to avoiding rejection immediately following submission. Editors can strike you out even without peer review if the justification is weak (Box C10.1).

The background is given in the first paragraph of the main manuscript text. Here you demonstrate that your topic has priority with respect to disease burden. The topic importance argument is typically advanced by giving the health problem prevalence. For uncommon conditions, the argument advanced can be based on a reduction in life quality and economic impact. The reports of authoritative bodies like the World Health Organisation or World Bank can be cited to back the argument along with the systematic reviews identified on the disease burden related to your topic. In the first paragraph of the introduction of your paper, among other citations, you include three authoritative body reports and three systematic reviews when you argue that *'migratory phenomenon has increased considerably .... providing vaccination services to this vulnerable population is crucial'*.

The justification for undertaking your review is provided in the second paragraph of the introduction section of the main manuscript text (Box C10.2). It states with references confidently that *'Previous systematic reviews have suggested that migrant groups generally experience lower immunization rates, but they have several limitations according to evidence synthesis quality assessment tools .... A comprehensive systematic review of the worldwide literature is required'* (citing AMSTAR-2 for quality assessment in the bibliography; see Box C1.3). Your submitted paper's justification, compared to others being considered at the same time by the journal, is likely to be taken seriously as it is backed by an overview of the previous evidence syntheses including their formal critical appraisal.

You follow the Step 2 writing tips: Your abstract and the main text methods section both give the resources searched with dates and search term combination, the use of any language or time restrictions, and the selection criteria matching explicitly the structured question. The main text results section provides the flow diagram of study search and selection ensuring that Figure 1 is titled fully stating *'Flow chart of study selection in the review of vaccination coverage among migrants'*, not just 'Study selection flow chart'. You also provide the funnel plot analysis in an online appendix when stating in the abstract that *'there was no funnel asymmetry'* and repeating the same in the main text at the end of the results section with *'there was no funnel asymmetry (Egger's test P = 0.051)'*. This detail must have impressed the journal editors and peer reviewers. In the discussion of the main manuscript text, where in the second paragraph you point out the strengths and limitations of your review, you are able to confidently state that your *'search without language and date restrictions yielded sufficient numbers of studies with a high number of participants to facilitate precise estimation of the association'*.

AMSTAR-2: The second version of AMSTAR (A MeaSurement Tool to Assess systematic Reviews), an instrument for evaluating the quality of systematic reviews (amstar.ca). See Case study 1, Box C1.3.

Step 3: Assessing study quality

Your abstract specifies the study design selected and provides the corresponding study quality assessment checklist, stating *'Study quality was assessed using Newcastle-Ottawa scale.... Overall risk of bias was low in 13 (30%), moderate in 22 (50%) and high in 9 (20%) studies'*. In the methods and results sections of the main manuscript text, you include the details of these quality assessments under separate subheadings. The studies selected are too many to tabulate their individual risk of bias

Bias either exaggerates or underestimates the 'true' effect of an intervention.

assessment within a succinct manuscript. You would have been able to include this in your Master's degree thesis but the journals tend to have quite tight word limits. So, you summarize the overall study quality assessment in a 100% stacked bar chart titled *'Figure 2. Quality assessment of the studies included in the review of vaccination coverage among migrants, using Newcastle-Ottawa scale (numbers in bars are numbers of studies)'* giving both the quality domains and the individual items. The table of individual study quality is included in an online appendix for completeness and transparency. In the discussion section, you cover the issues related to the risk of bias in the second paragraph concerning the review's strengths and limitations and conclude judiciously that in your view *'the [large] size of the summary result obtained and its precision provides protection against a spurious conclusion'.* Your thoroughness in risk of bias assessment is appreciated by the journal when it sends in its comments asking you for revisions.

> The **quality** of a study depends on the degree to which its design, conduct and analysis minimize **biases**.

Step 4: Summarizing the evidence

Your paper title already includes the term meta-analysis in the subtitle, and the abstract follows up on this giving details of the meta-analytic methods stating *'Data were synthesized pooling data from individual studies to generate summary odds ratio (OR) with 95% confidence interval (CI) using random effects model, assessing heterogeneity with I^2 statistic used'.* You follow up on this, reporting in the results subsection of the abstract that *'the odds of vaccination coverage among migrants were lower compared to non-migrants (7,375,184 participants; summary OR 0.50; 95% CI 0.37-0.66; I^2 99.9%)'* completing the picture concerning the evidence summary numerically.

> **Tables, figures and appendices:** Detailed titles permit them to stand alone and assist in understanding their contents without the need to refer to the abstract or the main text. Using the components of the structured question in the titles helps to link them up with the review's objectives. Full descriptions of the abbreviations need to be repeated even when provided in the abstract and the main text, using footnotes if required.

The above made explicit concerning your main findings upfront, all that remains is for you to give details in the main manuscript text. The methods section covers within the data synthesis subheading the meta-analytic methods explaining what data were statistically synthesized: *'From each study a single 2×2 table with the largest total sample, the largest number of doses, and the smallest difference in vaccine coverage was selected for meta-analysis to maximize precision and to produce the most conservative estimate of the association'.* The results section within quantitative data synthesis subheading provides a forest plot titled: *'Figure 3. Random-effects meta-analysis of vaccination coverage among migrants compared to non-migrants'.* This is backed by reporting of the 2×2 table data synthesized in your online appendix, economizing on the main manuscript word count while maintaining openness. This also permits data sharing for anyone else to replicate your data synthesis.

> **Data sharing:** Increasingly journals require review authors to give a statement specifying where the data reported in their review are available. Reviewers painstakingly extract data from the individual included studies for preparing detailed tables, figures and appendices. This automatically makes data available within their published review articles. In the interest of openness, there is a demand for reviewers to share their data spreadsheets electronically along with statistical codes and outputs.

Step 5: Interpreting the findings

Theoretically, the discussion section of the main manuscript text is expected to cover this Step narratively in a typical systematic review article. Not all systematic review papers formally draw on the strength of the evidence to generate inferences. The inferences are typically generated qualitatively by assessing the importance of outcomes, the various biases, the heterogeneity, the 95% confidence intervals, the funnel asymmetry, etc. The reviewer's commentary on these issues is often dispersed throughout the discussion section.

It is important to remember that interpretation accompanies factual information as it is presented throughout the article. At the beginning of the article, the abstract ends by presenting the conclusion that gives an answer to the review question and suggests its implications (for future research and practice). Thus, the abstract has to be front-loaded with interpretive information. Your conclusion is that *'Migrants are half as often vaccinated compared to non-migrants. Public health prevention programs need to prioritize vaccination equity, not just to protect migrants but also to protect the host communities'*. The first part of this conclusion is backed by the study quality assessments and data syntheses you have presented in the methods and results sections of the abstract. The second part concerning the implications of your findings would need elaboration in the discussion section.

To write the discussion section of the main manuscript text is a daunting task for novice review authors. Here we present some tricks that will permit you to take a stab at drafting the discussion without hesitation. The first thing to recognize is that the discussion need not be long; it should be clear and brief, following the structure provided in Box C10.3. The first paragraph should give the main findings, which should follow directly from the result subsection of the abstract. You just need to remove the numbers from the text in the abstract, replacing the statistics with appropriate descriptive words, e.g. odds ratio value of 0.50 can be described as odds reduction by half (Box C10.4).

In the next paragraph, the discussion section should cover strengths and limitations. As you conducted a sound review covering all the Steps described in this book, you take the liberty to claim that you *'followed a robust methodology so as to attempt to reduce the possibility of various forms of errors and biases'*. Following this grand opening, you can give the limitations in a way so as to explain what you did to deal with the potential weaknesses or what implications they might have. In one example in this Case, the limitation is provided with the inferential consequence that actually arises from it as follows: *'one perceived limitation of this study may be related to the fact that there is no universally accepted definition of a migrant at the international level. The lack of clarity about this general term leaves the interpretation somewhat open, generating issues in generalizability of our finding'.*

Box C10.3 Relation between the five systematic review Steps and the review manuscript structure

Manuscript structure (suggested length)	Review Steps	Comments, tips and tricks
Front matter and Abstract		
Title (12–15 words, 140 characters with spaces)	1	Ensure that the title contains as many components of the structured question as possible and the subtitle states the design.
Authors (>1; single author reviews are frowned upon)		Authorship ought to comply with the International Committee of Medical Journal Editors criteria (ICMJE, icmje.org). A formal honesty, accuracy and transparency guarantee is often required. It is a good idea to register your identity as an author (ORCID, orcid.org) and provide it to the journal.
Abstract (250 words) Use a structured abstract with at least four subheadings: Objective, Methods, Results, and Conclusion.	1–5	Some journals may provide additional subheadings and may also be more flexible with word count. Editors read the abstract to make their initial assessment. It makes the first (and the last) impression. To avoid rejection, write this first and rewrite it several times to help make a good first impression!
Main manuscript text		
IMRaD (<3000 words: some journals may permit up to 4–5000 words)	1–5	IMRaD (Introduction, Methods, Results and Discussion) structure is typically used. The use of generosity with word count offered by some journals should only be rarely necessary.
Introduction (350 words; 3 paragraphs) Give disease prevalence, reduction in life quality, economic impact, etc. (first paragraph), and justification of your review in light of deficiencies of previous reviews (second paragraph), before repeating the objective from the abstract (third paragraph).	1 and 2	A paper is not a textbook chapter. The background needs to be brief. The first and second paragraphs establish the importance of your topic and the justification for undertaking the review. Editors use this information to determine if your submission should be given priority over other manuscripts they have in front of them. In Step 2, when you conduct your searches, take note of published reviews concerning prevalence, reduction in life quality, economic impact, etc. to demonstrate documented disease burden. Assess existing reviews using a quality assessment checklist, e.g. AMSTAR-2 or ROBIS, to describe their weaknesses.

(Continued)

Manuscript structure (suggested length)	Review Steps	Comments, tips and tricks
Methods, Results (total 1650 words, split in around half for each; 3 subsections each) Give methods and results separately in subsections, each under subheadings to cover search and selection, quality assessment and data synthesis.	2–4	Follow a reporting guideline. Describe registration details. The methods and results subsections should be complementary covering study search and selection, data extraction and study quality assessment, and data synthesis. Patient and public involvement may be described in a separate methods subsection if required. Ensure that methods and results in the abstract match those reported in the main text.
Discussion (1000 words; 4 or 5 paragraphs) Give main findings, strengths and limitations, interpretation of findings and their implications for practice and research before drawing the conclusion. Some journals may offer the opportunity to write the discussion with subheadings.	1–5	The summary of major findings should match the results given in the abstract. Strengths and limitations can be drawn from the assessment of the review's quality in light of the critical appraisal points at the end of each of the five Steps in this book. Interpretation of findings can compare the review's results with those of previously published reviews (cited in the second paragraph of the introduction). Implications should be judiciously inferred and the conclusion should sing from the same hymn sheet as that in the abstract.
End matter		
Acknowledgements		Those who contributed to the review, but did not sufficiently meet authorship criteria, are named here. Obtain and retain written permission to be acknowledged by them.
Conflict of interest		A formal disclosure is mandatory and it may be submitted using an ICMJE form.
Bibliography	2	Ensure compliance with authors' instructions. If there are limits to the permitted number of references, you can always provide the references to the included and excluded studies in an appendix.
Tables, figures and appendices	2–4	Tables and figures will be incorporated into the main text following acceptance of the manuscript.

After these deliberations, you discuss your findings comparing them with those of other similar published reviews. Here your effort concerning the identification of previous reviews during Steps 1 and 2 while undertaking prospective registration and searching will come in handy. The references you boldly deployed in the justification paragraph of the introduction section in the main text can be redeployed for comparative interpretation (Box C10.4). In the introduction, you used the weakness of

Box C10.4 Relation between the review's abstract, the introduction section of its main text and its discussion section

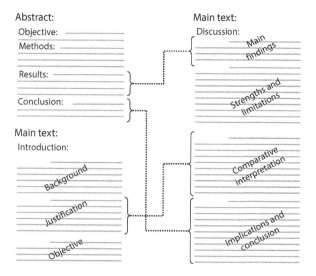

Abstract, Introduction and Discussion in the published paper

Abstract – results: 'Overall risk of bias was low in 13 (30%), moderate in 22 (50%) and high in 9 (20%) studies.... the odds of vaccination coverage among migrants were lower compared to non-migrants (7,375,184 participants; summary OR 0.50; 95% CI 0.37-0.66; I^2 99.9%)'.

Introduction – justification: 'Previous systematic reviews have suggested that migrant groups generally experience lower immunization rates,[13-15] but they have several limitations .... One of the reviews[14] applied language restrictions, risking overlooking relevant publications. Other reviews had geographical limitations, in one focusing on Europe[13] and in another on three low-income and middle-income countries'.[15]

Abstract – conclusion: 'Migrants are half as often vaccinated compared to non-migrants. Public health prevention programs need to prioritize vaccination equity, not just to protect migrants but also to protect the host communities'.

Discussion – main findings: 'The quality of the included studies was diverse, predominantly moderate.... High level of heterogeneity was found in the pooled results .... Our findings showed that migrants were half as often vaccinated compared to non-migrants'.

Discussion – comparative interpretation: 'The results of our meta-analysis are in accordance generally with the previously published narrative reviews.[13-15] Moreover, we were able to quantify the extent to which migrant groups experience lower immunization rates than native-born groups in the evidence collated without geographic restriction'. [note the reuse of the same superscripted references]

Discussion – conclusion: '.... migrants are significantly less often vaccinated compared to non-migrants, and public health prevention programs need to prioritize vaccination equity'.

See structured question in Box C10.2.

*Text reproduced based on Semergen, 2022; **48**: 96–105, doi:10.1016/j.semerg.2021.10.008.*

the previous reviews to justify the need for the review you undertook. Now you can use the same references this time comparing your findings with the results reported in the previous reviews and describing what your review adds to what is already known. You also insert a statement about the advance your work brought about as follows: *'Thus our review provides the current best quantitative evidence synthesis'*.

Finally, you conclude by giving implications of your findings. The conclusion is bound within the provisos placed taking into account the risk of publication bias, clinical and methodological heterogeneity, and statistical precision of the findings among other features. These were covered throughout your discussion. Your discussion mirrored the conclusion reached in the abstract (Box C10.4) and you emphasized in the penultimate paragraph leading to the conclusion that vaccinating migrants is *'something that will be crucial for the benefit of the entire population'*. The conclusion could be the last paragraph of the discussion section or it could be written under a separate heading if the guidelines of your chosen journal ask you to do so.

Resolution of scenario

Writing a systematic review article that will be accepted for publication by a peer-reviewed journal is not an easy task. Most Master's degree students who conduct high-quality systematic reviews will find it difficult to compress their thesis into a manuscript for publication. A review-based thesis would have taken much time and effort to complete. This Case study has demonstrated with a real example of a Master's degree student undertaking her first review project that it is possible for new reviewers to become published authors. Using this book, they can prepare a manuscript that can convince referees and editors to publish their very first review as an article in a medical journal.

The manuscript carefully drafted as outlined above was assessed by the journal to be suitable for publication after revisions. The student responded to comments given by the referees in a manner satisfactory to editors. The citation of the review undertaken in the Master's degree thesis in this Case study appeared in various publicly available databases. Its PubMed record is as follows:

- Vaccination coverage among migrants: A systematic review and meta-analysis. *Semergen* 2022; **48**: 96–105, doi:10.1016/j.semerg.2021.10.008. (PMID: 35101341)

Glossary

This glossary uses information from the publications listed in the Suggested Reading.

Absolute risk reduction (ARR)   *see* **Risk difference (RD)**.

Accuracy measure   A statistic for summarizing the accuracy with which a test predicts a diagnosis. There are three commonly used sets of accuracy measures for binary tests: sensitivity and specificity; positive and negative predictive values; and likelihood ratios. All these measures are paired. Single measures of accuracy are seldom used with the exception of the diagnostic odds ratio.

Adverse effect   It is an undesirable and unintended harmful or unpleasant reaction resulting from an intervention. It often predicts hazards from its future administration and warrants prevention or specific treatment or alteration or withdrawal of the intervention.

AGREE II   The second version of AGREE (Appraisal of Guidelines for REsearch and Evaluation), an instrument for evaluating the quality and reporting of guidelines (agreetrust.org/agree-ii).

AMSTAR-2   The second version of AMSTAR (A MeaSurement Tool to Assess systematic Reviews), an instrument for evaluating the quality of systematic reviews (amstar.ca). *Also see* **ROBIS**.

Applicability of findings   *See* **External validity**.

Attrition bias (exclusion bias)   Systematic differences between study groups caused by exclusion or dropout of subjects (e.g. because of side effects of intervention) from the study. Intention-to-treat analysis in combination with appropriate sensitivity analyses including all subjects can protect against this bias. *Also see* **Intention-to-treat (ITT) analysis** and **Withdrawals**.

Baseline risk   The frequency of outcome in a population without intervention. In randomized trials, it is the rate of the outcome in the control group of participants who may receive no treatment or placebo. It is related to the severity of underlying disease and prognostic features. A good prognosis is associated with low baseline risk while a poor prognosis is associated with a high baseline risk of undesirable outcomes. Baseline risk is important for determining how many will likely benefit most from an intervention. *Also see* **Number needed to treat (NNT)**.

BEME   An international collaboration (Best Evidence Medical and health professions Education) committed to the development of evidence-informed education in the health professions (bemecollaboration.org).

Bias (systematic error)   A tendency for results to depart systematically, either lower or higher, from the 'true' results. Bias either exaggerates or underestimates the 'true' effect of an intervention or exposure. It may arise due to several reasons, e.g. errors in the design and conduct of a study. This may lead to systematic differences in comparison groups (selection bias), differences in care or exposure to factors other than the intervention of interest (performance bias), differences in assessment of outcomes (measurement bias), withdrawals or exclusions of people entered into the study (attrition bias), etc. Studies with unbiased results are said to be internally valid. *Also see* **Random error**.

Binary data   Measurement where the data have one of two alternatives, e.g. the patient is either alive or dead, the test result is either positive or negative, etc.

Bivariate model   A statistical method for generating summary estimates of test accuracy. It adjusts for the correlation that might exist between test sensitivity and specificity.

Blinding (masking)   Blinding keeps the study participants, caregivers, researchers and outcome assessors ignorant about the interventions to which the subjects have been allocated in a study. In single-blind studies, only the subjects are ignorant about interventions, whilst in double-blind studies both the participants and caregivers or researchers are blind. Outcome assessors can often be blinded even when participants and caregivers can't be. Blinding protects against performance bias and detection bias, and it may contribute to adequate allocation concealment during randomization. *Also see* **Randomization**.

Boolean logic   Boolean logic (named after George Boole) refers to the logical relationship among search terms. Boolean operators AND, OR and NOT are used during literature searches to include or exclude certain citations from electronic databases. They are also used in Internet search engines.

Case–control study   A comparative observational study where participants/patients with the outcome (cases) and those without the outcome (controls) are compared for their prior intervention or exposure rates.

Clinical trial   A loosely defined term generally means to describe a study to evaluate the efficacy and effectiveness of interventions. This term encompasses study designs ranging from randomized controlled trials to uncontrolled observations of a few cases.

Clinical practice guideline   *See* **Guideline**.

Cochrane Collaboration   An international not-for-profit organization that aims to help with informed decision-making about healthcare by preparing, maintaining and improving the accessibility of systematic reviews of interventions (cochranelibrary.org). The major product of the Collaboration is the Cochrane Database of Systematic Reviews, which is part of the Cochrane Library. Those who prepare Cochrane Reviews are mostly healthcare professionals who volunteer to work in one of more than 40 Collaborative Review Groups (CRGs). Each CRG has a coordinator and an editorial team to oversee the quality of its reviews. The activities of the Collaboration are directed by an elected Steering Group and are supported by staff in Cochrane Centres worldwide. *Also see* **RevMan**.

Cohort study   A comparative observational study where participants with an intervention or exposure (*not* allocated by the researcher) are followed up to examine the difference in outcomes compared to a control group, e.g. those receiving no care.

Comparative study   A study where the effect of an intervention or exposure is assessed using comparison groups. This can be a randomized controlled trial, a cohort study, a case-control study, etc.

Confidence interval (CI)   The range within which the 'true' value of a measurement (e.g. effect of an intervention) is expected to lie in a population with a given degree of certainty. Conventionally, 95% confidence intervals are used. For binary data, the width of the confidence interval is related to the sample size and the numbers with the outcome within the comparison groups. *Also see* **Precision of effect**, **Standard error** *and* **Variance**.

Confounding   A situation in studies where the effect of an intervention on an outcome is distorted due to the association of the outcome with another factor, the confounding variable, which can prevent or cause the outcome independent of the intervention and is also associated with the intervention. It occurs when groups being compared are different with respect to important factors other than the interventions or exposures under investigation. Adjustment for confounding requires stratified or multivariable analysis. *Also see* **Randomization**.

Continuous data   Measurement on a continuous scale such as height, weight, blood pressure, etc. For continuous data, the effect is often expressed in terms of the mean difference. *Also see* **Effect size (ES)**.

Control event rate (CER)   The proportion of subjects in the control group in whom an event or outcome is observed in a defined time period.

Controlled clinical trial   A loosely defined term to describe a prospective comparative study for assessing the effectiveness of interventions (regardless of whether randomization is used or not). Watch out for indiscriminate use of this ambiguous term in reviews. It is also a MeSH in the Medline database.

Core outcomes   These are a minimum set of critical and important outcomes on which there is consensus that they directly measure what is clinically relevant. Systematic reviews are used to create a long list of outcomes which is then reduced to a core outcomes set through surveys collating evaluations of patients and practitioners. *Also see* **Outcome**.

Cost-effectiveness analysis   *See* **Economic evaluation** and **Efficiency**.

Critical appraisal   Transparent evaluation of medical literature, whether primary studies or systematic reviews, for their (internal) validity, precision and applicability (external validity). Appraisal concerning (internal) validity evaluates study quality or risk of bias. *Also see* **Quality of a study**, **Precision** *and* **External validity**.

Design (study design)   A description of the manner in which participants are assembled and followed up in a study to gather the data required to test a hypothesis. It is important to define the study designs suitable for inclusion in a review when formulating structured questions. *Also see* **PICO(D)**, **Participants**, **Intervention** and **Outcome**.

Diagnostic odds ratio   The ratio of the likelihood ratio for a positive test result to the likelihood ratio for a negative test result. It provides a single measure of accuracy. *Also see* **Accuracy measure**.

Diary keeping   A qualitative research method, usually an addition to questionnaire or interview data, where participants record experiences and emotions contemporaneously. It can be free form, where people write what they want to, or structured, where they have specific questions to answer or topics to write about.

Dose–response   A dose–response relationship (sometimes also called biological gradient) demonstrates that at higher doses the strength of association between exposure and outcome is increased.

Economic evaluation (e.g. cost-effectiveness analysis)   A study that takes into account both the clinical effectiveness and the costs of alternative interventions to address the question of how to achieve an optimal clinical outcome at the least cost. The term cost-effectiveness analysis is often used synonymously, but this is a misnomer. A full economic evaluation considers both clinical and cost outcomes, whereas a partial evaluation may only consider costs without regard to clinical outcomes.

Effect (effect measure, treatment effect, estimate of effect, effect size)   Effect is the observed association between interventions and outcomes or a statistic to summarize the strength of the observed association. The statistic could be a relative risk, odds ratio, risk difference, or number needed to treat for binary data; a mean difference, or standardized mean difference for continuous data; or a hazard ratio for survival data. The effect has a point estimate and a confidence interval. The term *individual effect* is often used to describe effects observed in individual studies included in a review. The term *summary effect* is used to describe the effect generated by pooling individual effects in a meta-analysis.

Effect modification   It occurs when a factor influences the effect of the intervention under study, e.g. age may modify responsiveness to treatment.

Effect size (ES)   This term is sometimes used for an effect measure for continuous data. *Also see* **Effect measure**.

Effectiveness   The extent to which an intervention (therapy, prevention, diagnosis, screening, education, social care, etc.) produces a beneficial outcome in the routine setting. Unlike efficacy, it seeks to address the question: Does an intervention work under ordinary day-to-day circumstances? Effectiveness trials tend to be pragmatic with adequate sample sizes, intention-to-treat analyses and an emphasis on generalizability when defining participant selection criteria.

Efficacy   The extent to which an intervention can produce a beneficial outcome under ideal circumstances. Efficacy trials tend to be small in sample size, with analyses focused on determining the effect in patients who are fully compliant and with narrowly defined participant selection criteria.

Efficiency   The extent to which the balance between inputs (costs) and outputs (outcomes) of interventions represents value for money. It addresses the question of whether clinical outcomes are maximized for the given input costs. *Also see* **Economic evaluation**.

Evidence-based medicine (EBM)   The conscientious, explicit and judicious use of current best evidence in making decisions about the care of individual patients. It involves the process of systematically finding, appraising and using contemporaneous research findings as the basis for clinical decisions. Evidence-based practice (EBP) is a related term. Both EBM and EBP follow four steps: formulate a clear clinical question from a patient's problem; search the literature for relevant clinical articles; evaluate (critically appraise) the evidence for its validity and usefulness; and implement useful findings in clinical practice, taking account of patients' preferences and caregivers' experience. Another related term is evidence-based healthcare, which is an extension of the principles of EBM to all professions associated with healthcare, including purchasing and management. Systematic reviews provide powerful evidence to support all forms of EBM.

Evidence synthesis   A systematic approach to collating relevant evidence to address a research question. The questions may be narrow or broad. Typical evidence syntheses are systematic reviews and meta-analyses of narrow questions, e.g. determining the effect of a single intervention. Broad questions, e.g. comparison of multiple interventions for the same condition, are addressed in umbrella reviews, network meta-analyses and guidelines. *Also see* **Review, Systematic review, Meta-analysis, Umbrella review, Network meta-analysis** and **Guideline**.

Experimental event rate (EER)   The proportion of participants in the experimental group in whom an event or outcome is observed in a specified time period.

Experimental study   A comparative study in which decisions concerning the allocation of participants or patients to different interventions are under the control of the researcher, e.g. randomized controlled trial.

Exposure   A factor (including interventions) which is thought to be associated with the development or prevention of an outcome.

External validity (generalizability, applicability)   The extent to which the effects observed in a study can be expected to apply in routine clinical practice, i.e. to people who did not participate in the study. *Also see* **Validity (internal validity)**.

Fabrication   Making up data and using them as if genuine.

Falsification   Manipulating data in a way that they are inaccurately represented.

Fixed effect model   A statistical model for combining results of individual studies, which assumes that the effect is truly constant in all the populations studied. Thus, only within-study variation is taken to influence the uncertainty of the summary effect and it produces narrower confidence intervals than the random effects model. *Also see* **Random effects model**.

Focus group   A qualitative research method. The collection of qualitative data using a group interview on a topic. Usually 6–12 participants are involved, and they can be used to gauge issues of importance. *Also see* **Interview**.

Forest plot   A graphical display of individual effects observed in studies included in a systematic review along with the summary effect, if meta-analysis is used.

Funnel plot   A scatter plot of effects observed in individual studies included in a systematic review against some measure of study information, e.g. study size, the inverse of variance, etc. It is used in the exploration for the risk of publication and related biases.

Generalization   The extent to which findings of a qualitative research study are consistent with findings of similar studies, adding to the understanding of a phenomenon. Within qualitative research, the aim is not to extrapolate to wider populations, so this term should not be confused with the terms External validity and Generalizability.

Generalizability   *See* **External validity**. *Also see* **Generalization**.

GRADE   The Grading of Recommendations Assessment, Development and Evaluation (GRADE) working group is an informal collaboration that aims to develop a comprehensive methodology for assessing the strength of the evidence collated in systematic reviews and for generating recommendations from evidence in guidelines (gradeworkinggroup.org).

GRIPP   Guidance or checklist for reporting involvement of patients and the public in health and social care research including in systematic review articles (*BMJ* 2017; **358**: j3453. doi: https://doi.org/10.1136/bmj.j3453).

Guidelines   Statements that aim to assist practitioners and patients in making decisions about specific clinical situations. They often, but not always, use evidence from systematic reviews. *Also see* **Living guidelines**.

Hazard ratio   An effect measure for survival data, which compares the survival experience of two groups exposed to different interventions.

Health technology assessment (HTA)   Health technology includes any method used by those working in health services to promote health, to screen, diagnose, prevent and treat disease, and to improve rehabilitation and long-term care. HTA considers the effectiveness, appropriateness, costs and broader impact of interventions using both primary research and systematic reviews.

Heterogeneity/homogeneity   The degree to which the effects among individual studies being systematically reviewed are similar (homogeneity) or different (heterogeneity). This may be observed graphically by examining the variation in individual effects (both point estimates and confidence intervals) in a Forest plot. Quantitatively, statistical tests of heterogeneity/homogeneity may be used to determine if the observed variation in effects is greater than that expected due to the play of chance alone. For making a clinical judgement about heterogeneity, one might look at the differences between populations, interventions and outcomes of studies.

Homogeneity   *See* **Heterogeneity**.

I² statistic   It is a statistic for assessment of heterogeneity during study synthesis. Ranging from 0% to 100%, it gives the percentage of total variation across studies due to heterogeneity.

IMRaD   An acronym that refers to the headings used in the main manuscript text, i.e. I-Introduction, M-Methods, R-Results, a-and, D-Discussion, when writing a review paper for publication.

Individual participant data meta-analysis   A meta-analysis that uses raw data collected in the primary studies to produce a summary result. *Also see* **Meta-analysis**.

Intention-to-treat (ITT) analysis   An analysis where subjects are analysed according to their initial group allocation, independent of whether they dropped out or not, fully complied with the intervention or not, or crossed over and received alternative interventions. A true ITT analysis includes an outcome (whether observed or estimated) for all patients. *Also see* **Attrition bias** and **Sensitivity analysis**.

Integrative review   Also called mixed methods systematic reviews, these reviews collate evidence generated using different methods (study designs) aiming to bring together both quantitative and qualitative data on the same topic.

Internal validity   *See* **Validity**.

Intervention   A therapeutic or preventative regimen, e.g. a drug, an operative procedure, a dietary supplement, an educational leaflet, a test (followed by a treatment), etc. undertaken with the aim of improving health outcomes. In a randomized trial, the effect of an intervention is the comparison of outcomes between two groups, one with the intervention and the other without (e.g. a placebo or another control intervention).

Interview   A qualitative research method. It involves questioning people about their views or experience of a phenomenon or event. Can range from structured, where each participant is asked the same questions, to unstructured, which consists of a list of broad areas to be covered, the exact format of each interview being determined as it progresses. *Also see* **Focus group**.

Inverse of variance   *See* **Variance**.

Kirkpatrick hierarchy   A classification of medical educational outcomes to capture the impact of educational interventions. It has various levels: 1a: Participation or completion captures attendance at and views on the learning experience, e.g. course evaluation; 1b: Modification of attitudes captures change in attitudes or perceptions, e.g. subjective reaction or satisfaction of participants with course, difference between pre- and post-course attitude questionnaire; 2: Modification of knowledge or skills captures change knowledge or skills, e.g. difference in scores from pre- to post-course; 3: Health professional's behaviour captures the transfer of learning to the workplace or integration of new knowledge and skills leading to modification of behaviour or performance, e.g. difference in performance after the teaching evidenced by more evidence-based prescribing and more frequent attendance at journal club; and 4: Change in delivery of care and health outcomes captures changes in the delivery of care attributable to the educational programme with or without assessments of improvement in the health outcomes and well-being of patients as a direct result of teaching, e.g. audit of practice showing greater compliance with evidence-based criteria.

Likelihood ratio (LR)   It is the ratio of the probability of a positive (or negative) test result in subjects with the disease to the probability of the same test result in subjects without the disease. The LR indicates how much a given test result raises (if positive) or lowers (if negative) the probability of having the disease. With a positive test result, an LR+ >1 increases the probability that the disease will be present. The greater the LR+, the larger the increase in the probability of the disease and the more clinically useful the test result. With a negative test result, an LR– <1 decreases the probability that the disease is present: the smaller the LR–, the larger the decrease in the probability of disease and the more clinically useful the test result.

Living guideline   A guideline linked to a living systematic review. Its statements are continually updated incorporating new evidence as soon as it becomes available. *Also see* **Living systematic review**.

Living systematic review   A systematic review continually updated after its completion so that the review remains current. This approach incorporates new evidence into the review as soon as it becomes available. *Also see* **Systematic review** and **Review**.

MARS   A guideline on Meta-Analytic Reporting Standards (*J Bus Psychol* 2013; **28**: 123–43. doi: 10.1007/s10869-013-9300-2). *Also see* **PRISMA**

Mean difference   The difference between the means (i.e. the average values) of two groups of measurements on a continuous scale. *Also see* **Effect and Standardized mean difference (SMD)**.

Measurement bias (detection bias, ascertainment bias)   Systematic differences between groups in how outcomes are assessed in a study. Blinding of study subjects and outcome assessors protects against this bias.

MeSH   Medical Subject Heading. A controlled term used in the Medline database to index citations. Other electronic bibliographic databases frequently use MeSH-like terms.

Meta-analysis   A statistical technique for combining (pooling) the results of a number of studies addressing the same question to produce a summary result. The large majority of meta-analyses summarize aggregate data reported in the published articles included in a systematic review evaluating the effect of an intervention. *Also see* **Systematic review** and **Individual participant data meta-analysis**.

Meta-regression   A regression model with effect estimates of individual studies (usually weighted according to their size) as the dependent variable and one or various study characteristics as independent variables. It searches for the influence of study characteristics on the size of effects observed in a systematic review. *Also see* **Multivariable analysis**.

Metasynthesis   The amalgamation of the results of a group of qualitative studies on the same or a related issue. Included studies can be evaluated and the findings combined. This is achieved from reviewing the published data and not from meta-analysing data.

Mixed methods systematic review   *See* **Integrative review**.

MOOSE   A reporting guideline for Meta-analyses Of Observational Studies in Epidemiology (*JAMA* 2000; **283(15)**: 2008–2012. doi:10.1001/jama.283.15.2008).

Multivariable analysis (multivariable model)   An analysis that relates some independent or explanatory or predictor variables (X_1, X_2, ...) to a dependent or outcome variable (Y) through a mathematical model such as $Y = \beta_0 + \beta_1X_1 + \beta_2X_2 + \cdots$, where Y is the outcome variable; β_0 is the intercept term; and β_1, β_2, ... are the regression coefficients indicating the impact of the independent variables X_1, X_2, ... on the dependent variable Y. The coefficient is interpreted as the change in the outcome variable associated with a one-unit change in the independent variable and provides a measure of association or effect. The multivariable analysis is used to adjust for confounding, e.g. by including confounding factors along with the intervention (or exposure) as the independent variables in the model. This way the effect of the intervention (or exposure) on the outcome can be estimated while adjusting for the confounding effect of other factors. *Also see* **Confounding**.

Negative predictive value   The proportion of subjects who test negative and who truly do not have the disease.

Network meta-analysis   A meta-analytic technique that may be used in systematic reviews addressing broad questions comparing multiple interventions for the treatment of the same condition. The term network refers to the direct and indirect comparisons of interventions which become available when the effects of individual interventions are collated in a single review. Take, for example, a review of trials in which some compare head-to-head treatment A with treatment B and others compare head-to-head treatment C with B. Even if there are no trials comparing A with C directly, with network meta-analysis we can compute through an indirect comparison a relative effect for A *versus* C using B as the common comparator. After making these direct and indirect (as well as mixed, i.e. pooling both direct and indirect effects for the same treatment pair when available) comparisons, network meta-analysis can produce a ranking of treatments according to their relative effectiveness. *Also see* **Systematic review, Umbrella review** and **Meta-analysis**.

Normal distribution   A frequency distribution that is symmetrical around the mean and bell shaped (also called Gaussian distribution).

NOS   The Newcastle-Ottawa Scale, an instrument for assessing the quality of non-randomized studies in systematic reviews (ohri.ca/Programs/clinical_epidemiology/oxford.asp). *Also see* **ROBINS-I**.

Null hypothesis   The hypothesis put forward when carrying out significance tests that states that there is no difference between groups in a study. For example, statistically, we discover that an intervention is effective by rejecting the null hypothesis that outcomes do not differ between the experimental and the control group. *Also see* ***p*-value**.

Number needed to harm (NNH)   It is the number of patients who need to be treated for one additional patient to experience an episode of harm (adverse effect, complication, etc.). It is computed in the same manner as NNT.

Number needed to treat (NNT)   An effect measure for binary data. It is the number of patients who need to be treated to prevent one undesirable outcome. In an individual study, it is the inverse of risk difference (RD). In a systematic review, it is computed using baseline risk and a measure of relative effect (relative risk, odds ratio). It is a clinically intuitive measure of the impact of a treatment.

Observational study   Research studies in which interventions, exposures and outcomes are merely observed with or without control groups. These could be cohort studies, case-control studies, cross-sectional studies, etc.

Odds   The ratio of the number of participants with an outcome to the number without the outcome in a group. Thus, if out of 100 subjects, 30 had the outcome (and 70 did not), the odds would be 30/70 or 0.42. *Also see* **Risk**.

Odds ratio (OR)   An effect measure for binary data. It is the ratio of odds of an event or outcome in the experimental group to the odds of an outcome in the control group. An OR of 1 indicates no difference between comparison groups. For undesirable outcomes, an OR that is <1 indicates that the intervention is effective in reducing the odds of that outcome. *Also see* **Relative risk**.

ORCID   The Open Researcher and Contributor ID is one of the platforms that provides a unique identifier for researchers (orcid.org).

Outcome   The changes in health status that arise from interventions or exposure. The results of such changes are used to estimate the effect. Clinically relevant critical and important outcomes are crucial for decision-making. *Also see* **Core outcomes** and **Surrogate outcomes**.

Overview   *See* **Umbrella review**.

***p*-value (statistical significance)**   The probability, given a null hypothesis, that the observed effects or more extreme effects in a study could have occurred due to play of chance. In an effectiveness study, it is the probability of finding an effect by chance as unusual as, or more unusual than, the one calculated, given that the null hypothesis is correct. Conventionally, a *p*-value of <5% (i.e. $p <$ 0.05) has been regarded as statistically significant. This threshold, however, should never be allowed to become a straightjacket. When statistical tests have low power, e.g. tests for heterogeneity, a less stringent threshold (e.g. $p < 0.1$ or < 0.2) may be used. Conversely, when there is a risk of spurious significance, e.g. multiple testing in subgroup analysis, a more stringent threshold (e.g. $p < 0.01$) may be used. When interpreting the significance of effects, *p*-values should always be used in conjunction with confidence intervals (CI). *Also see* **Confidence interval (CI)**.

Participants   Individuals taking part in a study. It is important to define their characteristics when formulating structured questions. *Also see* **PICO(D), Intervention, Outcome** and **Design**.

Patient and public involvement   Evidence syntheses carried out with the input of lay members of the public to improve their relevance and overall review quality. *Also see* **GRIPP**.

Performance bias   Systematic differences in the care provided to the study subjects other than the interventions being evaluated. Blinding of carers and subjects and standardization of the care plan can protect against this bias.

Phenomenon   An occurrence or a fact. Phenomenon is often used as a generic term for the object of a qualitative research study.

PICO(D)   An acronym used in formulating structured questions for evaluation of the effectiveness of interventions. P stands for participants, I for intervention, C for control and O for outcomes. PICO sometimes appears with a D added to represent study design. The acronym requires substantial adaptation for other question types, e.g. in test accuracy evaluations it does not readily provide for index tests and reference standards. *Also see* **Participants, Intervention, Outcome** and **Design**.

Plagiarism   Presenting written text as original when it is an identical copy of the text that is previously published.

Point estimate of effect   The observed value of the effect of an intervention among the subjects in a study sample. *Also see* **Confidence interval (CI)**.

Positive predictive value   The proportion of subjects who test positive and who truly have the disease.

Post-test probability of disease   An estimate of the probability of disease in light of the information obtained from testing. With accurate tests, the post-test estimates of probabilities change substantially from pre-test estimates. In this way, a positive test result may help to rule in disease and a negative test result may help to rule out disease.

Power   The ability to demonstrate an association when one exists. The ability to reject the null hypothesis when it is indeed false. Power is related to sample size and the number of outcomes in the comparison groups. The larger the sample size, the more the power, and the lower is the risk that a possible association could be missed.

Precision (specificity) of a search   The proportion of relevant studies identified by a search strategy expressed as a percentage of all studies (relevant and irrelevant) identified by that method. It describes the ability of a search to exclude irrelevant studies. *Also see* **Sensitivity of a search**.

Precision of effect   The width of the confidence interval reflects the magnitude of imprecision in effect estimation. *Also see* **Confidence interval (CI)**, **Standard error** *and* **Variance**.

Pre-test probability of disease   An estimate of the probability of disease before tests are carried out. It is usually estimated as the prevalence of disease in a given setting (e.g. community, primary care, secondary care, hospital, etc.). Sometimes, when such information is not available, it may have to be estimated.

PRISMA   A reporting guideline for systematic reviews, meta-analyses and their protocols focusing on reviews evaluating the effects of interventions using randomized trials (prisma-statement.org).

PROSPERO   A database of systematic reviews that have been prospectively registered prior to commencing the review (www.crd.york.ac.uk/prospero).

Publication bias   Arises when the likelihood of publication of a study is related to the significance of its results. For example, a study is less likely to be published if it finds an intervention ineffective. Reviewers should make all efforts to identify such negative studies; otherwise, their inferences about the value of intervention will be biased. Funnel plots may be used to explore the risk of publication and related biases.

QUADAS-2   The second version of QUADAS (a QUality Assessment tool for Diagnostic Accuracy Studies), an instrument for the evaluation of the quality of test accuracy studies (bristol.ac.uk/population-health-sciences/projects/quadas/quadas-2).

Qualitative research   Research concerned with the subjective world that offers insight into social, emotional and experiential phenomena in health and social care. Including findings from qualitative research may enhance the quality and salience of reviews.

Quality of a qualitative research study   The quality of a qualitative research study depends on the degree to which its design, conduct and analysis are trustworthy. Trustworthiness consists of several concepts including credibility, dependability, transferability and confirmability.

Quality of a study (methodological quality)   The degree to which a study (a primary study or a systematic review) minimizes biases. Features related to the design, the conduct and the statistical analysis of the study can be used to measure quality. This assessment determines the (internal) validity of the results. *Also see* **Risk of bias assessment**.

Quasi-experimental (quasi-randomized) study   A term sometimes used to describe a study where the allocation of subjects to different groups is controlled by the researcher, like in an experimental study, but the method falls short of genuine randomization (and allocation concealment), e.g. by using the date of birth or even-odd days.

QUIPS   QUality In Prognosis Studies tool to assess the risk of bias in studies of prognostic factors (*Ann Intern Med* 2013; **158**: 280–6. doi: 10.7326/0003-4819-158-4-201302190-00009).

Random effects model   A statistical model for combining the results of studies that allows for variation in the effect among the populations studied. Thus, both within-study variation and between-study variation are included in the assessment of the uncertainty of results. *Also see* **Fixed effect model**.

Random error (sampling error)   Error due to the play of chance that occurs when a sample of participants is selected to represent a population. *Also see* **Systematic error** or **Bias**.

Randomization (with allocation concealment)   Randomization is the allocation of study subjects to two or more alternative groups using a chance procedure, such as computer-generated random numbers, to generate a sequence for allocation. It ensures that subjects have a pre-specified (very often an equal) chance of being allocated to one of two or more interventions. In this way, the groups are likely to be balanced for known as well as unknown and unmeasured confounding variables. Concealment of the allocation sequence until the time of allocation to groups is essential for protection against selection bias. Foreknowledge of group allocation leaves the decision to recruit the subject open to manipulation by researchers and study subjects themselves. Allocation concealment is almost always possible even when blinding is not. Randomization alone without concealment does *not* protect against selection bias.

Randomized controlled trial (RCT)   A comparative study with random allocation (with allocation concealment) of subjects to interventions, and follow-up to examine differences in outcomes between the various groups.

Rapid systematic review   A review undertaken over a short time frame while attempting to maintain scientific rigour. Beware that quality may be compromised in such reviews. *Also see* **Systematic review** and **Meta-analysis**.

Relative risk (RR) (risk ratio, rate ratio)   An effect measure for binary data. It is the ratio of risk in the experimental group to the risk in the control group. An RR of 1 indicates no difference between comparison groups. For undesirable outcomes, an RR that is <1 indicates that the intervention is effective in reducing the risk of that outcome. *Also see* **Odds ratio**.

Research integrity   Compliance with ethical and professional principles, standards and practices by individuals or institutions in research.

Review   An article that summarizes the evidence contained in a number of different individual studies and draws conclusions about their findings. It may or may not be systematic. *Also see* **Systematic review** and **Meta-analysis**.

Review of reviews   See **Umbrella review**.

RevMan   The Cochrane Collaboration's software for review management and meta-analysis. *Also see* **Cochrane collaboration**.

Risk (proportion or rate)   The proportion of subjects in a group who are observed to have an outcome. Thus, if out of 100 subjects, 30 had the outcome, the risk (rate of outcome) would be 30/100 or 0.30. *Also see* **Odds**.

Risk difference (RD) (absolute risk reduction, rate difference)   An effect measure for binary data. In a comparative study, it is the difference in event rates between two groups. The inverse of RD produces the number needed to treat (NNT). *Also see* **Number needed to treat**.

Risk of bias assessment   An assessment that determines the (internal) validity of the results of a study (a primary study or a systematic review). *Also see* **Quality of a study**.

ROB-2   Version 2 of an instrument for assessing the Risk Of Bias in randomized trials (methods. cochrane.org/risk-bias-2).

ROBINS-I   An instrument for assessing the Risk Of Bias In Non-randomized Studies of Interventions (methods.cochrane.org/methods-cochrane/robins-i-tool). *Also see* **NOS**.

ROBIS   An instrument for assessing the Risk Of Bias In Systematic reviews (bristol.ac.uk/population-health-sciences/projects/robis/robis-tool). *Also see* **AMSTAR-2**.

Sample   Subjects or participants selected for a study from a much larger group or population.

Scoping review   A systematic review but without a clearly formulated question. *Also see* **Review** and **Systematic review**.

Selection bias (allocation bias)   Systematic differences in prognosis and/or therapeutic sensitivity at baseline between study groups. Randomization (with concealed allocation) of a large number of patients protects against this bias.

Sensitivity (recall) of a search   The proportion of relevant studies identified by a search strategy expressed as a percentage of all relevant studies on a given topic. It describes the comprehensiveness of a search method, i.e. its ability to identify all relevant studies on a given topic. Highly sensitive strategies tend to have low levels of specificity (precision) and *vice versa*. *Also see* **Precision of a search**.

Sensitivity (true positive rate) of a test   The proportion of those people who really have the disease and who are correctly identified as such.

Sensitivity analysis   Repetition of an analysis under different assumptions to examine the impact of these assumptions on the results. In systematic reviews, when there is poor reporting in individual studies, authors of primary studies should be asked to provide missing and unclear information. However, this is not always possible and reviewers often have to make assumptions about methods and data, and they may impute missing information. In this situation, sensitivity analysis should be carried out by involving a re-analysis of the review's findings, taking into account the uncertainty in the methods and the data. This helps to determine if the inferences of a systematic review change due to these uncertainties. In a primary study, there may be withdrawals, so sensitivity analysis may involve repeating the analysis imputing the best or worst outcome for the missing observations or carrying forward the last outcome assessment. *Also see* **Intention-to-treat analysis** and **Withdrawals.**

Specificity (true negative rate) of a test   The proportion of those subjects who really do not have the disease and who are correctly identified as being disease free.

SRQR   A guideline on Standards for Reporting Qualitative Research (*Acad Med* 2014; **89**: 1245–51. doi: 10.1097/ACM.0000000000000388). *Also see* **Quality of a qualitative research study.**

Standard deviation   A statistical measure of the dispersion of the individual measurements obtained from a sample of participants. *Also see* **Standard error.**

Standard error   A statistical measure of the precision of an estimation made using a sample of participants. It represents the uncertainty around the estimation of any statistical parameter whether it be a measure of central tendency like mean or effect size (like risk ratio for a group comparison). The higher the sample size, the smaller the standard error and the higher the dispersion of individual data points, the higher the standard error. Its squared value is also known as the variance of estimation. *Also see* **Confidence interval (CI), Precision of effect** and **Variance.**

Standardized mean difference (SMD)   Standardized difference in means is an effect measure for continuous data where studies have measured an outcome using different scales (e.g. pain may be measured in a variety of ways or assessment of depression on a variety of scales). In order to summarize such studies, it is necessary to standardize the results into a uniform scale. The mean difference is divided by an estimate of the within-group variance to produce a standardized value without any units. *Also see* **Effect**   (erroneously called standardized mean difference).

Strength of evidence   The strength of evidence describes the extent to which we can be confident that the estimate of an observed effect, i.e. the measure of association between interventions and outcomes obtained in the review, is correct for important questions.

Study design   *See* **Design.**

Subgroup analysis   Meta-analyses may be carried out in pre-specified subgroups of studies stratified according to differences in populations, interventions, outcomes and study designs. This allows reviewers to determine if the effects of an intervention vary between subgroups.

Summary receiver operating characteristics curve (SROC)   A method of summarizing the performance of a dichotomous test, pooling 2 × 2 tables from multiple studies or multiple cut-off points. It takes into account the relation between sensitivity and specificity among the individual studies by plotting the true positive rate (sensitivity) against the false positive rate (100-specificity).

Surrogate outcomes   A substitute for direct measures of how patients feel, what their function is or if they survive. They include physiological variables (e.g. blood pressure for stroke or HbA1c for diabetic complications) or measures of subclinical disease (e.g. degree of atherosclerosis on coronary angiography for future heart attack). To be valid, the surrogate must be statistically correlated with the clinically relevant outcome and capture the net effect of the intervention on outcomes. Many surrogates lack good evidence of validity. *Also see* **Core outcomes** and **Outcome**.

Systematic error   *See* **Bias**.

Systematic review (systematic overview)   Research that summarizes the evidence on a clearly formulated question using systematic and explicit methods to identify, select and appraise relevant primary studies and to extract, collate and report their findings. Following this process, it becomes a proper piece of research. It may or may not use statistical meta-analysis. *Also see* **Meta-analysis**.

Theme   An idea that is developed by the categorization of qualitative research data under its heading. The large quantities of data produced by the qualitative study are managed by the generation of themes and the coding of parts of the data to each theme. The perspectives of each research participant on each theme can then be compared and analysed.

Theory   Abstract knowledge or reasoning as a way of explaining social relations. Theory may influence research (deduction), or research may lead to the development of the theory (induction).

Trial   *See* **Clinical trial**.

Triangulation   Triangulation is the application and combination of several research methodologies in the study of the same phenomenon.

Umbrella review (reviews of reviews, overview)   A review of systematic reviews on a topic. An umbrella review may address a narrow question collating reviews on a single intervention or a broad question about the comparison of multiple interventions for the same condition. *Also see* **Review**, **Systematic review** and **Meta-analysis**.

Validity (internal validity)   The degree to which the results of a study are likely to approximate the 'truth' for the subjects recruited in a study, i.e. are the results free of bias? It refers to the integrity of the design and is a prerequisite for the applicability (external validity) of a study's findings. *Also see* **External validity**.

Variance   A statistical measure of variation measured in terms of the deviations of individual observations from the mean value. It quantifies the precision or the error in the estimation made using a sample of participants. The inverse of the variance of the observed individual effects is often used to weight studies in statistical analyses used in systematic reviews, e.g. meta-analysis, meta-regression and funnel plot analysis. This weighting makes the individual studies with lower variance (i.e. with less error in the estimation of individual effect) have more importance in the calculation of the pooled effect. *Also see* **Standard error** and **Precision of effect**.

Withdrawals   Participants or patients who do not fully comply with the intervention, crossover and receive an alternative intervention, choose to drop out or are lost to follow-up. If an adverse effect is the reason for withdrawal, this information can be used as an outcome measure. *Also see* **Attrition bias**, **Intention-to-treat analysis** and **Sensitivity analysis**.

Suggested reading

This book focuses on core information about systematic reviews. The intricacies of many of the advanced techniques described briefly in this book, e.g. methods of meta-analysis, meta-regression analysis, network meta-analysis, funnel plot analysis, etc., can be examined in the materials referenced here.

Aromataris E, Munn Z (eds). JBI Manual for Evidence Synthesis. JBI, 2020.

Available free at jbi-global-wiki.refined.site/space/MANUAL.

Available free at training.cochrane.org/handbook/current.

Available free at www.journalslibrary.nihr.ac.uk/hta/hta2190#/full-report.

Available free at www.york.ac.uk/crd/guidance/.

Egger M, Higgins JPT, Davey-Smith G (eds). Systematic Reviews in Health Care. Meta-analysis in Context. London: BMJ Publishing Group, 2022.

Higgins JPT, Thomas J (eds). Cochrane Handbook for Systematic Reviews of Interventions. Version 6.3. The Cochrane Collaboration, 2022.

Sutton AJ, Abrams KR, Jones DR *et al*. Systematic Reviews of Trials and other studies. Health Technology Assessment 1998; 2(19).

Systematic Reviews. CRD's guidance for undertaking reviews in health care. Centre for Reviews and Dissemination. York: University of York, 2009.

Index

Printed in the United States
by Baker & Taylor Publisher Services